BEYOND THE BEDSIDE

ALTERNATE CAREERS FOR THE REGISTERED NURSE

Dwayne Adams, RN, MS

ISBN 978-0-9850033-3-3

leverage your knowledge

THE NURSE
expert

a greater influence, impact & income

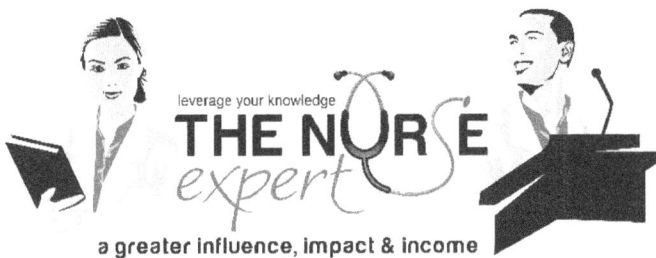

Beyond the Bedside, Alternate Careers for the Registered Nurse

Copyright © 2009 by Dwayne Adams, RN, MS

www.TheNurseExpert.com

ISBN 978-0-9850033-3-3

30 DAYS
of online RN Health Coach Training
ONLY $1 SPECIAL OFFER
www.HealthCoachNursingJobs.com
Use Special Code:BBBook

Dedication

This book is dedicated to all of those hard working nurses who have placed the lives of others above their own. It is for those who have shown the dedication and put in the time to help improve the lives of their patients. It is especially dedicated to those nurses who have been overworked, underpaid, and wish to continue their life of helping others, but want to find a new and different outlet to accomplish it.

Becoming a nurse is a demonstration of compassion, care and concern for the well-being of others. Being able to use the knowledge and skills that you have gained through nursing and turn them into a career as a RN Health Coach or other programs found at TheNurseExpert.com is a continuing way to extend your helping hand, and show your compassion.

"To accomplish great things, you must not only act, but also dream, not only plan, but also believe."

-Anatole France

Table of Contents

PREFACE

Being a bedside nurse can be a job that is rewarding as well as stressful and exhausting. Many registered nurses who have been in the field for a long time find their work slowly becoming less rewarding and more tiring and stressful. That, in fact, may be one of the reasons you are beginning to read this book right now, and it is important to remember that you are not alone in this thought.

The concept of this book was first developed as I myself was struggling to remember what it was that drew me into a nursing career. Amidst the problems and negative aspects of a high speed and intense working environment, I could not help but think that there was another way for me to utilize my skills to help others, as really that is a large motivation for most nurses. The more I looked into my outside options, the more I realized that I could touch other's lives in a positive manner through my work outside of a hospital or health care facility.

I found there are so many different options for registered nurses who wish to continue to use their knowledge and work experience but who also want to have more control over their career and working hours. When I found all of the opportunities available, I knew that I needed to share these with others who were in the same situation as I was. This book was created to share the knowledge that nurses who want to continue to help others, but are exhausted and burnt out from the stressful work of a bedside nurse, are able to find fulfilling and meaningful careers outside of this limited nursing field.

INTRODUCTION

All across America there are nurses who are trying to find the positives in their career and remember why it was they chose to go down the road that is registered nursing. The love for the career and what it entails has slowly started to fade because of the inevitable drawbacks of having a successful bedside nursing career. That something that drew them into being a nurse and putting everyone else before themselves has been lost in the jumble of everyday work problems and sacrifices they have made.

These thoughts riddle the minds of many registered nurses who have spent the majority of their working careers treating patients in hospitals and other health care facilities day in and day out. It is important to realize that many others share this thought, and that there are other ways to utilize your knowledge and skills. By picking up this book you have empowered yourself to make the best of your education and work experience, and take back control of your work life.

While there will always be certain problems within the nursing field, by no means do you need to limit yourself to having to deal with these issues. There are many different opportunities and possibilities for trained and registered nurses to find and take advantage of, especially in the case of Nurse Experts.

A Nurse Expert can be described as a nurse who wants to utilize their knowledge and experience in a way that can provide financial support. They are nurses who realize that their experiences and education can be used outside of the normal nursing field and can be leveraged and monetized. I teach entire lessons on this subject, more can be found by visiting www.TheNurseExpert.com Before we look further into the opportunities that are available to you, it is important that we first look at the problems that you, as a nurse, face within the nursing field.

Problems in the Nursing Field

Working as a registered nurse, you are very aware of the types of problems and issues that arise within your field. In many cases, you may not have actually sat down and listed the problems that you see, or perhaps you can quite define what they are, but you realize that something is just not quite right. More and more often registered nurses who work in bedside capacities are beginning to speak out more about the issues that they are noticing within their field. A field that they once believed to be full of job opportunity and potential, but is now falling short of their expectations and beliefs.

There are a number of common issues that nurses will see happening within the field of registered nursing. Some of these issues include:

- **Job Loss**. It is always said and believed that there are a number of nursing positions available and it will be easy to find work within the field. However, many registered nurses have begun to find that while there is a need for nurses, the job opportunities do not match that need. Unfortunately, the state of the health care industry within financial terms has greatly limited the availability of nursing jobs. While newscasts speak of nursing shortages, in many cases these shortages are unable to be filled because of financial reasons, even though the jobs are desperately needed. So while jobs are available, health care facilities are still having to lay off nurses in an effort to stay on budget, or cut back on spending, leaving the jobs unfilled, but still needed.

- **Leaving Nurses.** Part of the problem with budgetary cuts, or a decrease in facility spending, is the need to cut back on the workforce, and in many cases, this means a cut in the number of nursing positions. However, when these nurses leave the facility, the amount of work that needs to be done does not diminish but stays the same. This forces the remaining nurses to take on the workload and responsibility that used to be shared among many, but is now forced upon a few. As the stress and amount of work increases for the remaining nurses, they do not get paid for the extra work. The increase of work turns into an increase in stress and a decrease in job satisfaction. In many cases, nurses who remain after others leave end up also leaving that facility, or the field in general, because of the extreme stress and exhaustion from being overworked day to day.

- **Burned Out.** The two issues above regarding nurses' experience lead into and build up to this issue. Many nurses feel as though their work has burned them out. Their exhaustion and lack of consistent sleep due to stress takes a toll on their body and mind over time, burning them out. The more drained and tired they become, the less they remember why they entered this field in the first place, and it leaves them wanting to find a way out, but without the knowledge of how to do it, or what kind of work to seek.

- **Not enough staff.** For some nurses it is normal to show up for work and realize that you are vastly understaffed for your shift. This automatically means extra work and a more stressful work environment. Imagine the amount of stress that will build up by the end of the shift, when you are completing the work for four people with only two actually present. Unfortunately, this is becoming more and more normal as nursing shortages rise due to funding issues and financial stresses. So, while there are shortages, there is also no way to fill these jobs, no matter how many qualified candidates there are.

- **Work Schedule.** As a nurse, your work schedule is not determined by you but usually by the needs of the facility you are working for. This means that you need to be able to work for 12 hours or more in one shift at any time during the day or overnight. In many cases, nurses schedules are erratic and change on a week-to-week basis, making it hard to create a normal schedule at home and hard to spend time with family and friends. Many registered nurses feel that their schedule makes the rest of their life more difficult to plan for, and it brings stress from work into their personal life.

- **Vacations.** In many work places, the nursing staff is so understaffed already that taking vacation time off is a hassle and difficult to get. While nurses will earn vacation time throughout their work, it may become difficult or even impossible to get it approved as the need for the entire nursing staff is so high. This is especially difficult as bedside nursing is a career in which everyone needs time off to recharge and reboot in order to keep going.

These problems are common and can be seen in many different bedside nursing jobs; however, there are many more that nurses can attest to that are driving them to find other means of employment. Nurses feel as though the jobs that they went to school for and trained for are not fulfilling the promises that were made. In fact, many nurses feel underappreciated, underpaid and overworked. This does not have to be the case, and registered nurses can use their skills in a number of ways that will empower them as individuals and provide them with a stable living.

Nursing Careers are Changing

As you may have realized, the field of nursing careers is changing, and your sense of this may have been heightened after reading the information above. Some nurses have decided to step away from the changing field in order to find an outlet for their knowledge that is more fulfilling and works better for them. As the career of nursing begins to change, it is important to help nurses find a way to make the change a change for the better.

For many of the people who decided to become a nurse, it was for the joy and the satisfaction of being able to help people, to make a difference in their lives and to make a difference in the world. It is time to realize that as a registered nurse you can do this outside of the walls of a hospital or health care facility. You no longer have to rely on an employer to provide a job for you; take control of the situation and you will learn that you can make your own destiny within the nursing field. There are a number of opportunities for registered nurses looking beyond the bedside to start a business and to become their own boss.

The idea of a Nurse Expert fits perfectly along with the changes in nursing careers and the developments within technology and the use of the internet. A nurse expert is an individual who leverages the knowledge and experience they have gained in new ways as a way to create an income for themselves. The knowledge that you have gained as a nurse is extensive and multi-faceted, as a nurse expert, you learn how to use this knowledge to your advantage to create employment that can support you financially and a life that you are able to control.

Technology has made possible a number of opportunities for nurses looking to step away from the everyday turmoil of bedside nursing and become self-employed. You are already well equipped with the education, training, knowledge and experience; you just need to figure out how to put all of these traits to work for you. Through the use of computers, there is a large amount of job potential to work with. The internet allows you access to a number of people in all different walks of life, and you have knowledge to share.

Think about the potential that this audience provides you. If writing an e-book, or series of articles, you are fully able and capable of writing and self-publishing through the use of technology. The market for knowledge about health related issues is limitless and you are capable of creating a business for yourself in any number of arenas. Take advantage of the tools that are provided to you through technology and the internet. Utilize the skills you already have, and learn a new way of doing things, and you will be able to create and capitalize in the business world that is the center of the world today.

The New Method of Opportunity

It is easy to see that the changes in technology, added together with the changes in the nursing field and career opportunities, that there is an endless amount of new opportunities for registered nurses looking for alternative career choices. It is this knowledge that is turning many nurses away from the hospitals and corporations they work for in exchange for job potential and financial freedom.

It has been made clear in today's society that having jobs within corporations can be a risk, as financial crackdowns could mean quick job loss. The world has changed and job security is an issue that every American is faced with on a day to day basis. Working for others means facing that risk of being fired or having hours cut back. It is this information that lends itself to the idea of working for yourself and creating your own ending and success.

This has held especially true for me and my story of creating my own success. Through all of the negatives of the current economy and society, I was able to see the changes as something that can be taken advantage of, to see them as benefits, rather than negatives. Throughout this book, I hope that you are able to see these changes as benefits as well, and I hope they can be further illuminated by looking into my story.

My Story

I am a registered nurse who has spent over 10 years working within the nursing field as a bedside nurse. It was ten years of success filled with struggle and stress. Throughout my nursing career, it was clear to me that I always dreamt of starting my own business and working for myself.

There was something about being able to report to me and only me that made the idea of starting a business such an appealing one. Being able to call the shots and create the life that I wanted was something that seemed to be the perfect answer to my career issues.

I quickly realized that the dream of starting your own business is one that is not easily achieved. I tried a number of different times, in a number of different businesses and industries, and found myself repeatedly falling short and failing. With the hopes that continued education would help me succeed in these potential businesses, I sought out degrees in finance and marketing and kept trying.

At first, I didn't care what the business was, as long as I was working for myself and the business was successful. For me it was a case of trial and error; I learned about a number of different topics, tried many different business ideas, but in the end was having trouble being able to provide for my family as I continued to lose money in investments. Through all of this, I kept on chugging away, determined to learn from my mistakes and create a successful business.

Over time and through attending a number of different seminars focused on helping with writing, marketing and speaking I began to realize that my story of success was beginning to fall into place. One of the ideas that I had come up with, RNHealthCoach.com, had become a business that I was really succeeding in. In fact, before I even realized it, I had health coaches coming to me and asking my advice on a number of different topics.

It was then that I realized how many other people were in the same situation that I had been in: Nurses who were no longer happy with their bedside nursing careers, looking for a change, but unsure about how to make it happen. Through this realization, I created what is now known as the Nurse Expert brand.

I have been able to compile all of the information that I gained through my experience, my education, my trial and errors and my success and combine it into a program to help those who want to follow in my footsteps and create their own life and success. Through the Nurse Expert program, potential entrepreneurs will gain access to tools I have learned in my experiences including:

- Internet Marketing

- Professional Speaking and Writing

- Registered Nursing

- Public Relations

- Personal Coaching

When I was experiencing the failure and trial and error, I felt as though I was not even close to creating success, but instead the reality is quite different from that. Throughout that entire process, I was learning. I learned about many different areas of business, and in the end they all pointed me to the path that I am taking today, one that I am thankful for and grateful that it was created. It was the journey that taught me to overcome challenges and to push through the hard times to achieve a goal I so desperately wanted. It was the struggle that made me the successful entrepreneur I have become today.

What I have created with the Nurse Expert brand is a combination of every area that I learned from and educated myself in and created a business model that makes sense and works. It is a model that is aimed at making you a successful and self-employed individual. It allows you to benefit from the challenges that I overcame, without having to deal with the trial and error.

Through this brand, I have made available a new type of career for nurses looking for an alternative to bedside nursing careers. It will allow you to use your degree, your knowledge and your experience in a way that doesn't require you to work for a corporation or hospital. It will cover both the questions that arise from a small business owner's perspective as well as from the perspective of a registered nurse who wants to change careers and transition into a providing care away from the bedside.

It is Possible for You, Too!

What we have discussed should be a reason for you to get excited, even if it is just a little bit. This book provides a number of opportunities, and these opportunities are created and suited just for you!

Alternative options are available to you. Becoming a Nurse Expert is an option for each and every registered nurse that is out working hard hours and is fed up with being underappreciated, overworked and exhausted. Take the step towards creating a career that works for you; this is a field that every registered nurse can be successful in. Becoming a Nurse Expert can have a number of benefits for you, including:

- Control, be your own boss.

- Capability to explore something new.

- Continue to help others

- Use your education, knowledge and experience

- Using your creativity and expertise

- You dictate your work, life, and success

These are just a few of the many different possibilities and opportunities of a Nurse Expert. Everything that you are already equipped with allows you to create a life of success with every step. Every guide is available to you along with help, tips and other information at www.TheNurseExpert.com, which has program information.

Keep Reading!

This book has been created as a way to lay out the important aspects of providing care away from the bedside. It will allow you to find the alternatives to being a bedside registered nurse and the way to achieve success in these new opportunities. By reading and digesting the information contained in this book, you are providing yourself with the ability to create your own life, to be able to be in control of your work experience, your income potential, and your job opportunities. Each piece of information within this guide is putting you a step closer to being able to decide how you want to live your life.

RN HEALTH COACHING

The health care system is always changing and evolving, and as a Registered Nurse, it is important to stay on top of the curve. As the nursing industry changes, it may mean that nurses will have to seek out different ways to succeed with the skills that they have already acquired. Being a Registered Nurse has allowed you to gain the necessary skills and knowledge needed in order to help patients in the capacity of a Health Coach. Registered Nurse Health Coaching is an industry that is quickly growing and can help nurses develop their skill set and even potentially increase their income.

As the field of health coaching expands, it is important to get in this lucrative field at the ground floor. As individualized care is proving to be more and more needed in the health care industry, the area of health coaching is becoming more and more popular. As a registered nurse, you are distinctly prepared to be a part of this rapidly growing industry and career opportunity. Use your skills to bring a new sense of freedom to your work and find satisfaction in helping individuals make positive lifestyle changes that improve their quality of life.

What is Health Coaching?

Health coaching is a new profession and industry that is rapidly growing within the United States as well as across the globe. Health coaching is used as a way to help guide patients and individuals in approaching their health in a more positive and beneficial way. Health coaches will use a number of different methods to help their patients including setting goals, acknowledging obstacles, and creating support systems for achieving the goals. There are a number of benefits to the patient when a compatible relationship begins with a qualified health coach. It is a partnership that is based on accountability and focuses on achieving the specific health goals by working together.

Health coaching allows the coach and the individual a chance to identify the deeper issues and the specific habits and lifestyle of the patient and how it impacts an overall health plan. It allows for a much more individualized approach to health goals, such as weight loss or lower blood pressure and cholesterol. Because everyone has such a unique life and set of circumstances, each plan and set of goals will be different. Health coaching allows each individual and coach to create the plan that is best and most effective for them individually.

Importance of Health Coaching

What many people do not realize is just how much a person's lifestyle impacts both their everyday health and how they are able to deal with a variety of health issues they may experience. It has been found that many cases of disease or illness can be connected back to the individual's lifestyle and healthy or not so healthy behavior. It has been found that proper education and instruction when it comes to these health issues can have a major impact on the overall health of the patient and the ability to cope with the illness.

Some of the common diseases that have been found to be impacted by one's lifestyle and health habits include respiratory diseases, weight issues and diabetes, high blood pressure and cholesterol, and heart disease, as well as psychological issues such as anxiety and depression. These are diseases that are potentially preventable and can be remedied. Patients who are dealing with any of these issues can improve their quality of life through the use of a health coach.

Health coaching is so important because it can change lives. It is a chance to provide clients with personalized care tailored to help solve their individual problems through healthy life choices. Health coaching cannot only improve the overall health of the patient, but it can also help them to improve their overall quality of life.

The Need for RN Health Coaching

The state of the health within our nation is in crisis. We have one of the lowest average age expectancies, despite the fact that we pump the most amount of money into the health system in comparison to other countries. This makes it clear just how much change needs to happen within this system, as well as just how many people need to be provided with improved and more effective health care.

Some of the leading issues that have presented themselves in this country are that of obesity and health issues that relate or correspond to this. Obesity can be the cause of diabetes, high blood pressure and high cholesterol. In a prediction made by the World Health Organization, over 700 million people will be considered obese by 2015. Studies have even shown that over the next 20 years, the cost for obesity related problems and illnesses will make up over 15% of the overall US Health Care Costs.

It is clear that health coaching is a successful way to combat issues such as obesity and weight loss programs. The individualistic approach can have a larger impact on these members of society versus the current system for providing care to overweight patients. There is a distinct need for the type of care received when utilizing RN health coaching on an individual level for patients.

It is this clear need for an improved method of care that brings to light the business possibilities that you can achieve through the use of RN Health Coaching. It is necessary to meet the demands of the patients, and where there is demand, there needs to be adequate supply. There is much to be gained for both the patients as well as the providers of RN health coaching across the nation.

Common Areas of Health Coaching

Health coaching is used to help patients with a number of different health related problems, and focuses on the individuals' obstacles and goals. There are a number of health issues that truly require an individualistic approach, as they vary greatly from person to person. Creating a successful and healthy weight loss program is an aspect of health that can benefit greatly from the use of a health coach. The health coach has the chance to get to know the individual and their lifestyle in order to create a plan that is practical and effective for that specific person. Health coaches can help individuals reshape their life and their health for the better in many ways.

Another group that greatly benefits from the use of a health coach is those trying to break addictions, such as trying to quit smoking. This is a difficult process to go through and to be able to have a support system and a health coach creates a better chance of success. It allows the individual the chance to create a plan that is focused on their needs and success.

Areas Another area in which health coaching can have a large impact is the care of clients who are recuperating from injuries, accidents, or are in post-surgery recovery. Establishing a health coach relationship with a knowledgeable medical professional, such as a Registered Nurse, during these times of recovery can be an asset to having the best recovery possible. It allows the patient a chance to fully communicate how their recovery is affecting them on an individual level, and allows them access to a care plan that supports those individualistic needs.

Why is Health Coaching Successful?

There are a number of reasons why health coaching can be successful for both the patients and the coach. Most importantly, participating in health coaching is a decision that is agreeably entered into by both of you. When a patient wants to improve their quality of life, it allows for there to be much more success with being able to overcome their obstacles and achieve their goals.

Health coaching also provides the client and coach with accountability. This is a great way to motivate the patient into setting and reaching their goals. It is a way to provide both incentives and motivations to create a healthier lifestyle that is catered and fitted precisely to the individual. It is the synergy and partnership between the client and the coach that produces the successful results that can be seen through health coaching. As the relationship grows and strengthens, it is easier for clients to trust in the advice and benefit from it.

Many of the current health care initiatives are focused on those patients who are already sick and do not focus very heavily on the importance or prevention. Health coaching is a way to help prevent further medical or health related problems as it focuses on prevention. There is a need for a change within certain aspects of the health care system, and health coaching can be one of the solutions.

Why RN's are Qualified Health Coaches

A successful health coach is someone who has experience dealing with patients and a wealth of knowledge on a number of different topics. As a registered nurse, your career provides you with a great background in patient care and health information. Along with the knowledge and training that you have received over the years, you also have had experience on a day to day basis with dealing with a variety of patients and issues.

As a registered nurse, you have provided patients with a guide through their illness and recovery. On an everyday basis, you have demonstrated care and compassion along with trained communication ability in order to provide patients with all the necessary information. You are educated in how procedures work and are able to explain to patients clearly what to expect and how to deal with it. It is all of this and your ability to answer patients questions, fears and anxieties that have prepared you to be able to be an effective and helpful health coach for a number of different individuals.

Through the experiences of a registered nurse, you have been able to see first-hand what the consequences can be of an individual leading an unhealthy lifestyle. You have been given a unique glimpse into the immense need for a change in the day to day healthy behavior choices that people make, and you can make a difference. Each patient is unique and different, and your experiences show you just how much outside choices can affect their overall health and lifestyle.

It is all of your experiences and education that have prepared you to be able to offer patients and clients with specialized one-on-one treatment and advice through the partnership of a health care coach. Being able to have experienced the need for patients to have an individualized care plan based off their unique medical issues and concerns allows you to help create a better life for a number of individuals.

Possibilities of RN Health Coaching

Being a health coach as a registered nurse provides you with a number of new possibilities and benefits. As the health care system continues to struggle in the United States and abroad, it is important to find new ways to utilize all of the skills and knowledge you have amassed over the years. Health coaching allows you to use these experiences in a new way that will help to reach out to many people in need of individualized care.

Flexible Working Schedule

RN health coaching allows you to access a number of career benefits and different opportunities from increasing income to a more controlled working schedule. RN health coaching is growing quickly, and it allows you to set, schedule, and manage your own work, allowing you to become your own boss. One of the most attractive aspects of being able to work as a health coach is the chance to be an entrepreneur and truly be in charge of creating your own future. By allowing you to be in control of the amount of clients you take on as well as your schedule, it gives you freedom and flexibility to schedule work around your life.

Income Potential

RN health coaching provides the possibility to supplement your income in a way that can help provide financial stability as well as flexibility. There is an unlimited amount of income potential within the field of RN Health coaching; it is up to you how much you will be able to earn. You can utilize RN health coaching as a supplement to your other income, or even as the main and only source of your income.

How many patients you look to take on, as well as how much you charge, is directly related to how much income you will make. You are completely in control of your financial stability as a RN health coach. It even provides you with the opportunity to leave your current job and take on RN Health Coaching as your one and only full time employment.

There are a number of different ways that you can go about setting and achieving the type of income that you want. Let's take a look at different combinations of client hours per week and your charging rate that can get you to an income of around $50,000 per year.

Hourly Rate	Client Hours/Week	Monthly Income
$50	21	$4200
$75	14	$4200
$100	10.5	$4200

*Registered Nurse Salaries — Staff RNs working in the United States average a median base salary of $41,642. Half of all US RN's are expected to earn between $38,792 and $44,869. Source: Allied Physicians — Nurse salaries & Nursing salary surveys

Keeping in mind that the amount you work directly relates to your income potential, let's look at just how much you could make if you are pushing yourself and working more than 20 hours a week.

Hourly Rate	Client Hours/Week	Monthly Income	Annual Income
$50	35	$7000	$84,000
$75	35	$10,500	$126,000
$100	35	$14,000	$168,000

The income opportunity that presents itself through the possibility of this profession is an amazing chance to improve your quality of life. It allows you to be fully in control of how much you are making. It will ease the stress of waiting for your next paycheck, and it will allow you to plan for life's obstacles with more control and flexibility.

Individualized Care and Patient Success

RN Health coaching allows you to truly connect with each patient on an individual level. You are able to help and assist them in creating a lifestyle that will improve their quality of life and health. There is a great sense of reward when you see your clients improving their health and making healthy life choices. Being able to be a direct factor of that improvement leaves you with a great sense of accomplishment and shows the true impact you can have as a health coach.

Utilizing Existing Skills and Knowledge

All of the skills and knowledge that you have gained over your years of working as a registered nurse will relate directly to your experiences as a health coach. Your patient interaction and knowledge of symptoms, illnesses and healthy behavior choices provides you with all the necessary skills. Health coaching allows you a way to use your skills in a new and different industry that has an unlimited amount of potential. Unlike other job changes where you have to be retrained, health coaching is unique in that you already have all of the necessary skills.

My Experience in RN Health Coaching

I am a testament to the potential success that can be gained by registered nurses through RN health coaching. I have been successful in gaining clients through a network developed to assist RN's who are seeking to start their own health coaching business. Through the use of L.I.T.E. Therapeutics, creators of RNHealthCoach.com, I have been able to set up my own business and begin to create a business through the use of their resources and support.

I have had great success utilizing the marketing techniques in order to attract new clients and make a name for myself and my business. There is a large amount of individuals who need this type of individualized care, and as a RN I already had the skill set to help them; I just needed the support to create a business out of my knowledge and experience. RNHealthCoach.com provided this system of support and business knowledge to help me begin this experience.

How to Get Started with RN Health Coaching

Getting started with RN health coaching is not difficult; it simply requires you to have the proper support and knowledge on how to be successful in this area. There are a number of different ways to go about starting your career as a RN Health coach. As you are already equipped with the necessary skill set and experience when it comes to the coaching, the part that usually needs the most help is the business side of this career choice.

It is important to create a business and marketing plan that will help get your name out and attract potential customers. This is often the most difficult part for up and coming health coaches, as it is the part where they have the least amount of experience. There are successful services such as L.I.T.E. Therapeutics that provide a support system to help RN's establish and grow their business.

RN Health Coaching Resources and Support

Finding a support system and resources to utilize as a new and upcoming RN Health Coach is an important part of creating a successful business within this industry. While your knowledge and experience provide you with the ability to provide effective coaching to your patients, it is also important to remember the business side of becoming an entrepreneur. Having access to enough support and resources make a large difference in the success of a RN Health Coaching business.

www.HealthCoachNursingJobs.com is a great resource to use for RN Health Coaches looking for training as well as a number of necessary resources. It provides you with education as well as assistance in creating a successful Health Coaching business as a Registered Nurse. Along with this training and resource site for RN's looking to become health coaches, is the sister site, www.RNHealthCoach.com, which is geared towards consumers and clients looking for a qualified Health Coaches.

L.I.T.E. Therapeutics has provided me with a great sense of support and a number of different resources that have helped me to establish a good base of clientele and give my business just the type of jumpstart it needed to get going and become successful. It is these resources and the support provided that have allowed my business to grow as it has, and continues to do so.

Some of the resources and help that they provided me with to establish my success included qualified training on a monthly basis on client relations and marketing, among other topics. In addition, they also have a number of resources that are available to their members such as marketing strategies and tips, as well as a manual to success in starting your own RN Health Coach Business.

Chapter Review and Key Points to Remember

Making the decision to become a RN health coach is one that could improve your life as well as the lives of others. Throughout this chapter, we have discussed many different aspects within the business of Health Coaching, especially for registered nurses. It is an area that is growing rapidly and the time to get involved is now. There are a number of key points to remember when beginning to consider becoming a RN health coach.

Key Point - As a registered nurse you are already equipped with many of the skills and knowledge needed to be a successful health coach in a number of different areas. Through your job and patient care experience and your education, you are well prepared to step into this new area of individualized health care.

Key Point - RN health coaching is focused on individualized patient care. By being able to focus on individuals and creating personalized care plans, you are better able to aid in their success. This provides your patients with a higher quality of care and provides you with more job satisfaction as you see your patients improve through your hard work.

Key Point - You are your own boss when you start a health coaching business. This translates into you being able to have more flexibility with your work and career. RN Health Coaching allows you to have more freedom with your life, job and working hours. With flexible hours, you are able to cater your job around your life. It enables you to determine just how much time you work, and gives you control over your work schedule when life's obstacles step into the way, as they always seem to do.

Key Point - Your income potential through RN Health Coaching is limitless. Starting your own business enables you to create the life that you want for yourself. The amount of work that you do will correlate to your income potential. It allows you to be in charge of your life and allow you to determine how successful you want your business to be. Many RN Health Coaches end up making a considerable amount more working as their own boss than they were making as registered nurses working for a hospital or other health care provider.

The income opportunity that is available through this type of profession can greatly impact the quality of life and provide more freedom and flexibility for nurses who are used to working long shifts and crazy hours. A simple formula translates precisely the number of client hours you put in into the type of income you will be achieving. Being in control of your finances is a blessing that the majority of workers in America do not have the opportunity to reach. The possibilities for income increases are limitless when it comes to becoming a successful RN Health Coach in the health care system these days.

Key Point - Resources are readily available for you to utilize in order to improve the success of your business.

The RN Health Coaching websites such as www.HealthCoachNursingJobs.com are available for you to use for training resources as well as networking possibilities. Along with the consumer site, www.RNHealthCoach.com, which provides networking opportunities, you are provided with a number of resources to create a successful business.

Summary

RN health coaching is an area of health care that is emerging quickly as a way to deliver high quality care on a personalized and individual level. It allows for personal contact and care in a way that the client or patient may not receive through conventional health care options. RN health coaching is a beneficial industry for both the providers as well as the clients. It allows for the clients to receive better care and for the providers to connect with their patients on a personal level which provides more job satisfaction.

This type of care is so important for our nation because many people are not finding success in combating areas such as weight loss, diabetes and obesity. For many people the difference between achieving success and not achieving success is the difference between having a care plan that is personalized to them. The relationship between a coach and a client allows the coach to create a plan that will better suit each client individually.

Through the use of all of the provided resources and training through L.I.T.E. Therapeutics, Inc and their websites, www.HealthCoachNursingJobs.com www.RNHealthCoach.com & www.TheNurseExpert.com registered nurses looking to begin this business have all they need to get started.

The potential is limitless as far as income and job satisfaction are concerned, and countless lives can be touched through this work. It is an important type of care that is needed by many people throughout this country and the world.

For more information on becoming a RN Health Coach,
Visit: **www.HealthCoachNursingJobs.com**

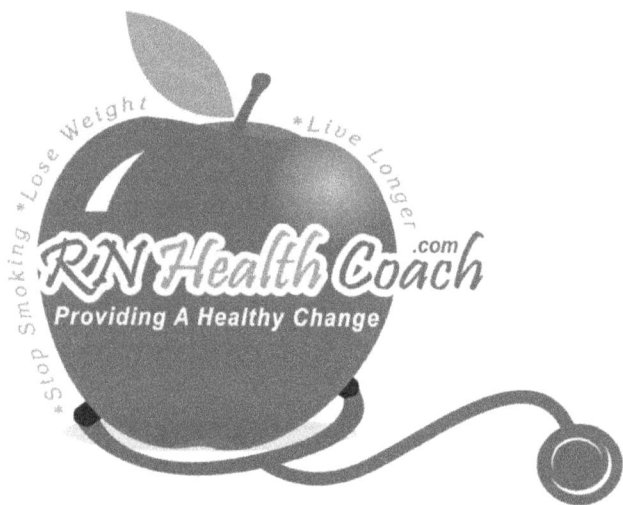

LEGAL NURSE CONSULTANT

Duties of a Legal Nurse Consultant

A Legal Nurse Consultant is a registered nurse that carries a level of expertise and specialized training in order to consult on issues relating to legal cases. Bridging the gap by properly informing and assisting attorneys, a Legal Nurse Consultant shares their knowledge on the health care system, while the attorney then applies such information to the legal issue at hand. A Legal Nurse Consultant will work as a part of the litigation team, but is not to be confused with the duties of a paralegal.

While a paralegal assists attorneys with various legal services and requires a different form of education, a Legal Nurse Consultant, or LNC, is actually a specialty practice of the nursing field, which does not require them to have a certain understanding of the legal system. While this knowledge is likely gained along the way, it is not required in order to have a successful career as a Legal Nurse Consultant. Instead, they use their area of expertise within the health care profession to educate and consult with clients on specific medical and nursing issues as they pertain to each case.

As a Legal Nurse Consultant, your goal should be to work as a liaison between attorneys, clients, and physicians. Some typical duties of a Legal Nurse Consultant may include the following:

• Performing assessments on hospital and nursing facilities

• Providing expert testimony in regards to duties and activities associated with healthcare and nursing

- Reviewing of various documents
- Preparing exhibits lists
- Interviewing healthcare professionals and witnesses
- Reporting illnesses and injuries
- Evaluating damages
- Identifying codes of practice
- Communicating with expert witness
- Examining medical records
- Completing research within the field using literature in order to deliver opinions
- Providing overall support during the discovery phase of the case, as well as during the actual trials
- Aiding in depositions or may possibly be deposed themselves

Ethics

The Code of Ethics and Conduct in which a Legal Nurse Consultant must follow are crucial. The following guidelines include how professional performance and behavior should be conducted within this particular field.

A Legal Nurse Consultant is not restricted by race, nationality, sex or sexual preference, age or social status. When performing any and all duties, these factors must be considered, understood, and respected. In no way should personal attitudes interfere with ones professional performance.

They should perform their duties as an expert or consultant while maintaining the highest level of integrity. This includes honesty, sincerity, and uprightness. Both a sacred and personal trust, a Legal Nurse Consultant must uphold these standards despite any difference in opinions. Never at any time will poor judgment, deceit, or deficiency in principles be tolerated.

Upon accepting assignments, a Legal Nurse Consultant should always use informed judgment, individual competence, and objectivity. They should not consult in matters in which they do not have appropriate experience or knowledge. They should also be sure to maintain personal conduct standards by abiding by all state and federal laws. In the event that a Legal Nurse Consultant becomes involved with illegal or unethical activities knowingly, public trust and confidence will be jeopardized.

Providing this professional service should be done with objectivity; meaning, free of both conflict of interest and any personal prejudice. Before taking on assignments, any possible interference must be recognized before acceptance.

Both privacy and confidentiality of the client should be protected by the Legal Nurse Consultant. Confidential material should be used discreetly. Any personal information of the client should not be used for personal gain of the consultant. The Legal Nursing Consultant will be held accountable and responsible upon acceptance of any case they take on Lastly, the consultant must maintain their professional nursing competence. Practice and standards should be current. The consultant must be a registered nurse and keep their nursing licenses current.

Qualifications Skills

If you are interested in this field of nursing, it is important for you to know what is expected in order to succeed in this career. The specialty practice of a Legal Nursing Consultant does have some education requirements, as well as skills that will allow the Legal Nurse Consultant to continue successfully within this career. Some skills that will be helpful include:

- Strong oral communication and written skills

   Great communication is a very important part when working alongside attorneys, when dealing with clients, and when talking with other healthcare experts. As a Legal Nurse Consultant, you should be able to take complex information and put it in understandable terms, which is why being able to communicate effectively and having strong writing skills is a must.

- Organization and analytical skills

   A Legal Nursing Consultant should also be extremely organized, as well as analytical. Since the information you work with is so complex, it needs to be analyzed and organized logically. This will help with the many tasks you will be completing including sorting medical records, developing a case strategy, making suggestions about which expert witnesses to use, and much more.

- Flexible

   It is important that a Legal Nurse Consultant is flexible and easy going. Sometimes you may need to deal with difficult patients when having to develop a plan for individuals who are withdrawn.

A LNC, however, should be able to provide support making stressful situations less intense and they do so successfully by being easy going and easy to work with.

- Strong Research Skills

  Strong research skills are very important and are something a LNC must possess. Specifically, internet research because you will need to be researching medical literature, various contact information, background checks, obtaining hard copies of journal articles, as well as medical text books, and much more. Ideal research skills will also save a lot of time, making the job of a Legal Nurse Consultant more effective.

- Persistency

  Dealing with rejection is part of the job of a Legal Nurse Consultant, so having the skill of persistency is going to be imperative. Going through research and medical records in search of important details pertaining to a case will certainly require one who is persistent.

Education

To become a Legal Nurse Consultant, the first step is to complete the formal requirements to become a Registered Nurse. A few options to accomplish this that include a 2-year associate's degree, a 3-year diploma that is hospital based, or a 4-year bachelor's degree. Some will further their education with a postgraduate degree such as a master's degree or a doctorate.

All nurses are also required to be properly licensed by the state in which they will work. Each state has a state nursing board that provides the proper licensing. Once this has been accomplished, work experience is the next step in becoming a Legal Nurse Consultant. This is important because it allows you to learn the specialty role of a LNC.

While there are many professional organizations that offer certification for this field of nursing, they are all voluntary in nature and are not mandatory requirements. In order to work as a LNC, holding a certificate is not a necessity. On that same note, it can be helpful in demonstrating your skills and knowledge within the specialty.

In short, the only 'must have' qualification to become a Legal Nurse Consultant is to be a Registered Nurse. While many will take extra measures to be competitive, such as obtaining certifications and learning more about the legal field, it is not a prerequisite.

Certifications

Although you are not required to gain a specific certification in the legal nurse consulting field, many will still do so to heighten their knowledge and advance their careers in this fast growing industry. There are many places to obtain your legal nurse consulting certification including online and local universities. If this is an option you choose to take, consider that many programs are not recognized by certain boards, such as the American Board of Nursing Specialties, also known as ABNS. So, although not required to function as a LNC successfully, you still may want to consider getting certified through a prestigious board.

The following includes a few options as to where you can obtain your Legal Nurse Consultant Certification:

-American Legal Nurse Consultant Certification Board (ALNCCB)

www.aalnc.org

* Accredited by the Accreditation Board for Specialty Nursing Certification (ABSNC)

-National Alliance of Certified Legal Nurse Consultants (NACLNC)

www.legalnurse.com

* Accredited by the American Nurses Credentialing Center's Commission on Accreditation

Employment

Legal Nurse Consultants will work with legal matters that have a medical angle. This includes:

- Healthcare licensure and investigations that are related

- Personal injuries

- Malpractice in the medical field

- Product liability

- Workers' compensation

- Risk management

- Toxic torts

A LNC has various options when it comes to employment. They can start their own business working as an Independent Contractor or work for a company that hires Legal Nurse Consultants. The types of companies that hire LNCs include:

- Insurance companies

- Defense or plaintiff attorneys

- Organizations that focus on health maintenance

- Hospitals and other medical facilities

- Private industries

- Government entities

Finding Employment

If you decide that you would like to work for a company as a Legal Nurse Consultant, guidance in finding that ideal job will be extremely helpful. While you will need to remain consistent and patient in your search, the following are some tips to help you along the way.

- Resume

  You're going to want to create a resume to impress. Some tips in doing so include highlighting both your positive points as well as your strengths. Keep your resume to three pages maximum. Be sure to use bullet points and consider keywords that are incorporated in online searches. It is suggested that you do not list hobbies.

- Job Boards

  Job boards are actually extremely popular and are frequently used by Human Resource Departments. Executives of law firms also observe job boards to find prospective candidates as well. Some of the more popular job boards include:

  - LawJobs.com

  - Monster.com

  - JobCircle.com

- CareerBuilder.com

- Beyond.com

- SimplyHired.com

- Indeed.com

- LegalNurseConsultantJobs.com

- Recruitment Agencies

  Another helpful resource in finding a Legal Nurse Consultant job is through recruitment agencies. There are many highly reputable agencies throughout the United States that allow you to register and upload your resume. Some of these include:

  - Spherion Staffing Services

  - Robert Half Legal

  - Davidson Staffing

  - Michael Page

  - Apple One

- Law Firms

  Another great option in finding employment is to go straight to the law firm. If you want to work as a Legal Nurse Consultant for an attorney, go directly to the source. The following are considered the top firms that employ Legal Nursing Consultants:

  - DLA Piper Rudnick Gray Cary

  - Baker & McKenzie

  - Sidley Austin Brown & Wood

  - Lewis Brisbois Bisgaard & Smith LLP

  - Latham & Watkins LLP

• Classifieds

Let's not forget that classifieds may also have job postings for those seeking to hire a Legal Nurse Consultant. Classifieds can be found in online newspapers, online job search sections on various websites, or classified sites where you submit and circulate your own ad. The following list includes great places to get started.

Online Newspaper Classifieds:

- New York Times
- Washington Post
- USA Today
- Classified Sites:

•

- FlipDog
- Craigslist
- eBay Classifieds
- Linkedin
- Oodle

- Ad Submittals:
- Craigslist
- City-Data

• Facebook

In your search, don't underestimate the power of Facebook. Here, you can socialize with not only other Legal Nurse Consultants, but with recruiters as well. Be sure to "like" these other Facebook members and join in their conversations. You never know if this will lead you to a job. Some of the conversations you may want to look into include:

- Get Legal Nurse Consultant Jobs Group

- USA Jobs Forever

- Discover Legal Jobs

- Compare Legal Jobs

• Email Alerts

Signing up for email alerts is important because it will allow you to be one step ahead of other job seekers. It could mean the difference between you getting the interview or the person who responded before you. There are many places in which you can register your information to then receive job alerts through your personal email. Some of the more popular ones include:

- Lawjobs.com

- NationJob.com

- Jobster.com

- CareerExposure.com

- CareerBuilder.com

- Associations

  Finding further information about being a Legal Nurse Consultant will also be helpful when it comes to your job search. To do this, you can contact various associations that apply to the industry. To name just a few:

  - American Association of Legal Nurse Consultants (AALNC)
    401 North Michigan Avenue
    Chicago, IL 60611
    (877) 402-2562
    http://www.aalnc.org

  - American Society of Legal Nurse Consultants
    4781 North Congress Avenue, Suite 184
    Boynton Beach, FL 33426
    (888) 336-3050
    http://www.aslnclegal.org

Private Nursing Practice

An increasingly common decision that nurses make is self-employment and maintaining their own Legal Nursing Consultant business. A private legal nursing practice allows you the freedom and ability to set your own hours, change locations if desired, and much more.

As with any other new business venture, the importance of planning before starting up your own business cannot be stressed enough. It is important that during this process, you dig deep within and ask yourself the hard questions.

It is going to be important to develop your own plan that starts with identifying your unique personal and professional vision. This means taking some time alone and giving careful thought to the important goals you have for your life.

Before making a decision, whether you will be self-employed or work for another company, it is important to visualize your ideal work life while considering things such as time and vacation flexibility, whether you desire to work alone or with others, whether you will require a support system and other issues. Remember, your personal life must be in line with your professional vision. If you fail to consider these aspects, the chances of achieving your goal will be greatly diminished. In short, do not rush through this important step in the process.

Equally important to the process of making such a decision are all the things required to actually set up and maintain the business. This is going to include things such as:

- Choosing a location

  You are going to need to make decisions about the location for your business. Most beginning entrepreneurs that need to save money on overhead look into alternative options for office space. You can also choose to work from home or if you would like your own office space for your practice, consider sharing office space (and expenses) with another professional until your business grows.

- Starting up operations

  Among the many things required to start up your business operations, you will need to open a bank account for your business. You may need financial funding. Bookkeeping, taxes and insurance are also other important matters that must be taken care of.

- Marketing

You will also need to invest in marketing materials such as business cards, a website, and more. Marketing is a 'must have' when it comes to starting any sort of business if you want to be successful. The good news is that there are several tools made available to help you along. For assistance with planned Health PR services, you can visit www.PRHealthCareCommunications.com or for SEO web marketing services, www.MediacalMarketingSEO.com will be very beneficial.

Although there are many other tasks needed in order for you to start up your own business that may seem daunting, you can achieve your business goals with both patience and planning.

Experienced Legal Nurse Consultants who have successfully started their own practices can offer several tips for those who are new to the industry. These tips include:

- Subcontracting

A great place to get started before starting your own business is with subcontracting. It will allow you to get your feet wet through networking with other Legal Nurse Consultants who belong to either chapter or national associations. This allows you to establish long lasting relationships.

When you subcontract for LNCs that are more seasoned, you can gain great advantages because they already have a rapport with their attorney clients. Since it is likely that a seasoned LNC has many cases, this will also assist in building your experience. You receive the benefit of having a mentor and coach, which will help to prepare you for the professionalism required to start your own business.

- Competition

  When you start your own legal nurse consulting business, you are going to want to be well aware of your competition. You are going to need to recognize that it does exist so that you can set yourself apart from it. Any business owner should know their weaknesses, strengths, and with both, have a well-developed plan on how to stand out in such a crowded field.

- Find and Use Tools for Success

  With the technology of the internet, we are now able to find a whole slew of resources that help us in the area we desire, and the same goes for those who choose to start their own business as a legal nurse assistant.

  Because there are so many resources available at our fingertips, it can be difficult to find the most effective tools. Whether you are trying to market, seeking to further your education, looking for guidance, or whatever the need, you can find the required help. The following resources are some that will be able to help you along in your business venture.

- The Pioneer of Legal Nursing

  Vickie Milazzo is known as the pioneer of legal nurse consulting and has been in the business since 1982. She offers a variety of useful tools and knowledge that pertain to the field including books, DVDs, blogs, courses, and much more. To explore what this industry leader has to offer you, whether you are self-employed or work for a company, visit LegalNurse.com.

- Marketing and PR Tools

  The best places to start when looking for ideal marketing and public relations tools is at these websites:

  PRHealthCareCommunications.com
  MedicalMarketingSEO.com.

  Having a website is going to be crucial to your success and in order to drive clients to your services; you are going to need to set up a website that incorporates search engine optimization. There is no question that you are going to have a lot of competition, but these tools will be able to assist in setting you apart and above the rest.

- Other Resources

  Keep in mind that there are many books that you can read to help get your Legal Nurse Consultant business off the ground. The best place to start is with The Nurse Expert Series, by Dwayne Adams, RN. The only way to become an expert is to learn from experts, and these books can guide you along the way.

Income Potential

For Legal Nurse Consultants who are independent contractors, they can charge anywhere from $60 per hour to $250 per hour. In some cases, even higher rates can be charged depending on the specialized duty. For example, if deposition preparation is required, or a court testimony is needed, a Legal Nurse Consultant can charge the client more.

On that same note, a Legal Nurse Consultant may consider charging hospitals less, about a range from $60 per hour to $80 per hour. This is because for a hospital to hire a full time Legal Nurse Consultant, it will cost them within that hourly range. Chances are they will not want to pay more when they could simply just hire someone full time to complete the same tasks.

A Legal Nurse Consultant who chooses to expand their career into more of the legal industry, can also charge more for their services. For example, a Registered Nurse can complete a two year associate's degree in paralegal work, enhancing their career, making them more specialized and allowing them to charge higher rates of up to $250 per hour. Some may obtain a degree in law, which justifies such a high hourly wage.

A Legal Nurse Consultant who is employed by a company will make an average of $125 to $150 per hour. They tend to make a little more than average versus Registered Nurses. While an RN makes an average of about $65,000 per year, a Legal Nurse Consultant will make an average of $80,000. This is because a LNC can work independently and charge more for their services.

In addition to working for a particular company, such as a law firm, a Legal Nurse Consultant may also receive various benefits such as health insurance, paid vacation, paid holidays, 401k plan, and so on.

Chapter Review and Key Points to Remember

By now, you have probably made your choice of whether or not you would like to pursue a career as a Legal Nurse Consultant. You may have even decided whether or not you want to start your own business or work for a company. Regardless, you should congratulate yourself for taking the first steps and following through with such a commitment to get the information you need.

Within this chapter, you have learned about the details of this career path. To review specifically what we covered, let's observe the key points.

As a Legal Nurse Consultant, it is important that you understand your duties and what will be required of you to complete your job successfully.

Key Point - In this chapter, you learned that a Legal Nurse Consultant will work as a liaison between attorneys, clients, and physicians. There are a variety of tasks that you will perform. Some of these include the evaluation of damages, interviewing healthcare professionals as well as witnesses, examining medical records, and much more.

Included in this chapter was information regarding ethics. Issues regarding discrimination based on culture, race, sex and other life choices were covered. As a Legal Nurse Consultant, the cases you work on should not be restricted by any of these issues.

Key Point - You, as a Legal Nurse Consultant, are responsible for following certain guidelines as to how you should be performing and behaving as a professional within this field.

We also reviewed the various education and skills that you should possess in order to be successful in your career.

Key Point - While there is no special degree to obtain in becoming a Legal Nurse Consultant, you are required to meet the formal requirements in becoming a Registered Nurse. You can choose to become certified, but it is not necessary. Certain skills that you should possess, that will help you in your career as a Legal Nurse Consultant, include strong oral communication and written skills, analytical and organizational skills, flexibility, research skills and persistency.

Your work will entail assisting with legal matters that include a medical angle.

Key Point - These duties include things such as investigations related to healthcare, personal injuries, malpractice, workers compensation, risk management, product liability, and toxic torts.

As a Legal Nurse Consultant, you can choose one of two options. You can either become employed for a company or become self-employed.

Key Point - Whether you decide to become a contractor or work for a company, the types of companies that will require your services include insurance companies, attorneys, organizations that focus on health maintenance, government entities, private industries, as well as hospitals and various other medical facilities.

Finding employment can be a difficult task, but with the help of tools as well as patience and consistency, you can find success in your search.

Key Point - Create your resume to be eye-catching, take advantage of job boards, use recruitment agencies to help in your search, contact law firms, search for options in classified ads, use social networking sites to help, such as Facebook.com, receive email alerts and lastly, contact associations.

If you decide that a private nursing practice is for you, just as with starting any business, you are going to have to consider many different aspects.

Key Point - While working from home can offer flexibility and many more benefits, you need to make careful decisions. Some decisions to consider include choosing a location, ideal start up operations, how to market, how to gain experience through subcontracting, knowing your competition, and finding and using the many available tools that can guide you to success.

Summary

Chances are you are reading this material because you have made the decision to start a career as a Legal Nurse Consultant. The next step is going to be determining your goals, whether you are going to further your education through obtaining a certificate, start your own business as a Legal Nurse Consultant, or begin your search for working alongside a company.

Regardless of which path you decide to take, remember to remain focused, as well as open to any new possibilities you will encounter. Also, remember that there is a wealth of information available to help guide you in your choice whether you seek to enhance your resume, start up your own business, or enhance your career.

Lastly, don't try to go it alone. Be sure to take advantage of all the resources and tools available to you. Do not be afraid to accept helpful advice and support to help you reach your goals in becoming a Legal Nurse Consultant. Always maintain confidence that you are a skilled professional fully up to the challenges and willing to do what it takes to be a Legal Nurse Consultant.

WORKSITE WELLNESS COACHING

It has become clear in the American culture, that the costs associated with health care is going to continue to rise until something is done to impact change. In fact, the current trend of rising costs is projected to continue to rise at a rate much faster than the general rate of inflation. With these numbers taken into consideration it is possible that the costs of healthcare could increase more than 10 percent per year, an astounding and troubling number.

In many cases, one of the main groups that is impacted by these numbers are employers who provide health care coverage and end up contributing a large amount of premium costs for individuals as well as their families. It is important that these businesses and employers, as well as their many employees, find ways to keep the costs down while still receiving high quality care. One of the ways to go about achieving this is through the use of worksite, or workplace, wellness.

There are a large number of benefits that can be achieved through the use of worksite wellness, and these benefits can impact both the employer and employees in many positive ways. While the idea of worksite wellness is not a new one, it is important to place renewed emphasis on the concept, especially in today's economy as well as within the current state of the nation's health care industry.

What Is Worksite Wellness?

The concept of worksite wellness is based around the implementation of a program within a workplace that works at providing employees with a number of tools to help improve their overall health and quality of life. Worksite wellness programs utilize a combination of health services such as educational opportunities, as well as activities that encourage or support the health of the employee both within the business environment as well as at home and beyond. Worksite wellness is also often referred to as workplace wellness or in many cases as corporate wellness.

Establishing a worksite wellness program at a business or organization can have a number of different benefits to both the employer and the employee and that is why they have become a popular option for many companies. Many companies across the United States offer these types of programs to their employees with a number of different goals in mind.

Why is Worksite Wellness Important?

The concept of worksite wellness is an important one for a variety of reasons. Most importantly, employers want to be able to provide their workers with not only a healthy and safe place to work, but they want to show them that they care about their well-being both inside and outside the workplace. Worksite wellness is an important part of creating a workforce that is happy, healthy and loyal to their company and employer.

Worksite wellness promotes a healthy workforce, which in turn translates to a number of positive benefits for both the employee and employer. Having healthy workers means having to deal with fewer employee absences, and creates a more productive set of workers. Decreased absences not only translates to more productivity for the company, but also translates to workers who do not have to miss out on a day of work to stay home sick, something that may create financial hardship. Worksite wellness provides employees with a sense that their employer has an invested interest in their health as well as the health of their families.

Goals of Worksite Wellness

There are a number of different goals of worksite wellness; however, there is one main overarching goal of the entire process and that is the increased health of the company or organization's workforce. Many worksite wellness programs are put into place by companies as a way to highlight the many ways that workers can take action to improve their own health and prevent a number of health issues that are common and likely to arise in many Americans. The majority of health issues that carry high health care costs are directly preventable through a number of different and easily achievable steps and measures.

Lower Health Care Costs through Prevention and Preventative Measures

One of the main goals of worksite wellness is to shine a light on the types of health care issues that can be directly prevented through education and knowledge about how to live and how to make health choices. When employees take advantage of the options offered through worksite wellness programs, they not only work towards improving their health, but also towards lowering their health care costs. Employees who lead healthy lifestyles and make healthy and fit choices generally have substantially lower health care costs, and much of that can be impacted by a well put together worksite wellness plan.

There have been a number of different studies done that show just how much the cost of health care is directly related to a number of risk factors as well as general health practices that individuals participate in. One of the main areas that have been looked into is the relationship between obesity and being overweight and health care costs.

It has been shown that an individual who is deemed to have an unhealthy Body Mass Index is almost four times more likely to be hospitalized than an individual who has a healthy Body Mass Index. In addition, it is common for those with an unhealthy BMI to have to have outpatient visits 2 or 3 times more often than those who are of a healthy weight and BMI. It is the extra hospitalization and general care of these individuals that translates directly into an increased cost of health care. In fact, the Kaiser Permanente Study in the Archives of Internal Medicine, Oct. 25, 2004, showed that the median annual health care costs of overweight individuals was 75 percent higher than those considered to be in the healthy weight group.

In addition, overweight workers cost upwards of $273 more each year when compared to workers who maintain a healthy weight. Further research also shows that obese workers, those with BMIs of 30 or more, cost upwards of $767 more each year than the group of workers who are considered to be at a healthy weight.

GM Study – Overweight and Healthcare Costs

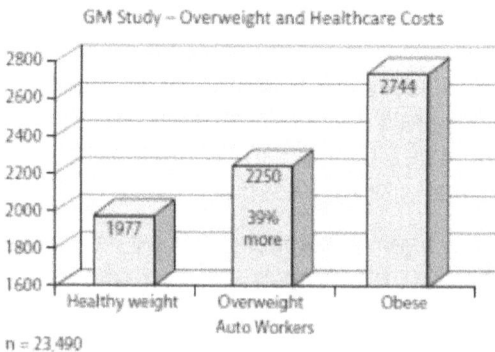

n = 23,490

Journal of Occupational and Environmental Medicine May 2004)

Employer Benefits of Worksite Wellness

Employers will directly benefit from putting in place a well-run worksite wellness program for their employees in a number of different ways. While the main goal and benefit is increased health of employees, this also comes with a number of additional benefits as well.

Help to Control the Cost of Health Care

Worksite wellness programs are a great way to work towards lowering the cost of providing health care for employees. Through a number of educational programs as well as activities provided to workers, employers are able to better promote healthy lifestyles and provide the opportunity for employees to utilize healthy options at work. When the overall health of employees is raised, the amount of associated health care costs for those employees goes down. With many of the most prevalent health issues preventable through education and positive health improvement programs, it is clear how a healthy employee would translate into lower health care costs. This not only lowers costs for the employer, but also for the employee.

Help to Attract and Retain High Quality Workers

Being able to not only attract, but to also retain, high quality workers is a task that many companies strive to achieve but also at times have a difficult time doing. Worksite wellness programs are a great way to show current and potential employees that the business they work for has a vested interest in their future, not only related to business, but to their overall health and well-being. It is a way to show employees that the company is willing to go the extra mile to ensure the highest quality of care for those who work for them. Being able to demonstrate to workers that they are an important part of the business is an important part to establishing and keeping a motivated and high quality workforce.

Increase Productivity and Decrease Work Absences

Increased productivity is something that every business strives for; however, many of these businesses fall short in creating increase productivity. One of the benefits of worksite wellness is that it is a great way to increase the productivity of your workforce. In fact, there have been many research studies done that show that a healthy workforce, both mentally and physically, will produce much higher productivity ratings than workforces who are not provided with healthy worksite wellness programs. While many programs are aimed at lowering health care costs, it has been found that the main impact of worksite wellness programs may actually be productivity instead of lower health care costs.

A workforce that is consistently healthy is more able to work productively, improve their method of working, and have a higher amount of energy and brain power to dedicate to their work. When they are supplied with the needed education and information to make their lives healthier it directly influences how productive they will be within the workplace as well as at home and in other capacities. This is especially true when much of the work is physically demanding, as those who are unfit are more likely to suffer from injury than those who are in shape. Loss of workers due to injury or bodily weariness is a large part of productivity and financial loss for a company or business.

Along with increased productivity, having healthy workers also means that they will likely need less days off due to illness or doctor's visits. This means that the company will experience less days when they are short a worker, which usually means decreased productivity or increased amount of work on fewer employees. This is something that not only benefits employers but also benefits employees as they will have to miss less days, which could possibly be without pay.

Increase the Corporate Image

There is no law or rule that forces companies to participate in worksite wellness programs. In fact, in many cases the main reason behind the participation of companies is to be a benefit to the employees who dedicate their time and effort to the business. Starting a worksite wellness program is a great way to show these employees that the company cares about their health, not just the work that they provide. Worksite wellness programs are a way to promote a corporate image that cares about employees, not just about the bottom line. It is a way to present the company in a positive light to employees as well as shareholders or potential business partners.

Improve Employee Moral and Loyalty

The morale and loyalty of employees is an important part of running a successful business. An important part of maintaining employee morale and loyalty is showing your employees that they matter past providing your business with work and knowledge, but that they matter as individuals and people as well. Worksite wellness programs allow your employees to see that you value them as a whole person, not just as a small part to the larger business model. Increased or improved morale and loyalty also translate to increased effort among employees and improved productivity.

Employee Benefits of Worksite Wellness

While the employer or company may be instituting worksite wellness programs for their benefit, it is clear that there are also many benefits for employees from these worksite wellness programs. With the goal of the programs being to improve employee health and overall well-being, the company and employees will realize a number of benefits as well.

Receive Better Health Care at Lower Costs

Worksite wellness programs are a great way to teach employees how to live lives that will help to promote overall health. These educational programs are a way to help employees decrease their health care costs simply because they are working at preventing potential health issues. Lowering their health care costs by being proactive about their health allows them to have increased amounts of money to spend on the things that their family wants or needs.

Learn to live a Healthier Lifestyle

These programs offered through worksite wellness are a way to learn and implement important health knowledge that otherwise employees may never have had access to. Knowing what the problems are and being able to alter a lifestyle to avoid these problems is the first step to a healthier nation. In addition, along with a healthier nation will come smaller health care costs. Learning to live a healthier lifestyle will not only affect the quality of work that one does, but will also affect the quality of life they have outside of work with their families and friends.

Reduce the Chance of having Major Health Problems

Many doctors agree that the biggest part of avoiding health problems and issues is having the knowledge needed to live a lifestyle that decreases one's chance of having these problems. This is the main goal of worksite wellness programs. Being able to educate employees on the most prevalent health issues of the day as well as what they are able to do in order to avoid these problems. Prevention is the key to maintaining a healthy life and being able to live longer without the presence of major health issues, and prevention comes through education and being in an environment conducive to healthy lifestyles.

How to Get Companies to Adopt a Worksite Wellness Plan

1. Stress Importance and Gain Support of Decision Maker

In order to create the want and need for this type of program in a business it is important to be able to stress the importance of these programs to the person in charge of making the decisions. Highlight all of the different benefits to both the business and employer as well as the employees of the business. It is important to show how much of an impact a plan like this could have on a business's strength and growth in productivity and employee morale and loyalty.

2. Discuss and Plan Budget

Implement a budget plan for the specific company's wellness program. It will be different for each company and it is important to be able to craft a program around the available funds. Use your knowledge of educational costs and determine what aspects to include in the budget and label the ones with the highest priority. It is important to know what amount of investment needs to be made in order to truly see a return on the money put into a worksite wellness program.

Research shows that companies who invest between $150 and $400 for every employee will see the most benefit and return on the investment. When beginning to discuss budgets with the individual in charge of making the decision, talk in terms of percentage of employee benefits, rather than in dollar amounts. This allows them to see how small of a portion of their benefit package can have a positive effect on the business.

3. Perform Health Risk Assessment

It is important to utilize a health risk assessment as a way to gage the current state of employee health and to know what the risks and interests of each employee currently is. Through the evaluation of a health risk assessment, you as a worksite wellness coach will be able to better prepare a plan that suits the individual company and the needs of their current employees. It allows you to be able to determine which programs will best benefit the company and employees. Health risk assessments also provide you with a method to measure the productiveness of the programs you are implementing from year to year.

For many companies starting out, offering worksite wellness and health risk assessment have a general participation level for the first year of only 30 percent. It is thought that at least a 70% participation rate is needed in order to have the most influential impact on the overall health of the employees. In order to achieve higher participation rates within the health risk assessments, it is a good idea to offer incentives along with participation in order to achieve the highest participation rate possible.

Health risk assessments allow you to determine the categories of risk that are applicable to certain businesses. There are generally three categories of risk when it comes to HRA's. Low risk (which measures between a 0-2), medium risk (which measures between a 3-4) and high risk (which measures as 5 and over). In addition, you need to consider the risk of existing disease.

Each assessment will lead to a different approach to what programs to offer to employees. High risk employees will benefit from risk reduction programs such as health coaching, as well as disease specific management programs for those with existing issues. Low risk employees will benefit from health promotion programs including options such as health screenings, newsletters and seminars which promote healthy behavior and lifestyle changes.

4. Perform Culture Survey

Assess the current culture within the corporate business and determine the changes that need to be made. It is sometimes simple and small changes that can be made that make a larger impact on the overall health and well-being of the workers. Look at the types of food offered in the cafeteria, the company's current smoking policy or if there are any incentives for participating in a wellness program.

5. Plan Interventions/Programs to be offered

Determining the types of programs and plans that should be offered can be partially determined by the Health Risk Assessment and the overall evaluation of current employees and their interests. Each company will have a unique set of interests that can be determined and changed by a number of factors. Creating a personalized plan for each business is the best way to help them succeed as well as see the return on investment for participating in worksite wellness programs.

Some of the common areas of concentration for worksite wellness programs range from simple newsletters and seminars, to more cooperative measures such as screenings and health coaching for individuals or groups. Below are some of the options that can be offered through a worksite wellness program.

a. Lifestyle Management/Health Coaching

These generally relate to the overall wellness of individuals and groups within the business or company. They are common among many employees and span over any type of company industry or workplace from physically labor intensive jobs to desk jobs.

i. Condition-Specific Weight Loss

Obesity and overweight employees have been shown to have a much higher health care cost when compared to workers that have what is considered a healthy weight. As obesity and overweight individuals continue to rise in this nation, this is an issue that is likely to affect a number of different workplaces.

ii. 8 Weeks to Wellness

General wellness programs such as '8 weeks to wellness' work at promoting general wellness and are beneficial to both high risk and low risk employees. They work at promoting general life changes that will help improve health through making healthy choices and learning what choices most impact one's health.

iii. Smoking Cessation

Even with the knowledge of how harmful smoking can be, it is still a main factor in the overall health of individuals in the workplace. While this may affect a smaller group of workers, it is still an important part of worksite wellness to promote, especially if it has a large presence in a specific company.

iv. Emotional Health & Mind Body

In many cases the factor of emotional health is looked past for more physical manifestations of health. However, it is not something that should be overlooked, as those with higher emotional and mental health are better workers and are more productive in their work capacity.

b. Disease Management

Identifying the need for disease management is an important part of workplace wellness programs. While it may not affect the majority of a workforce, it is the cause of a large portion of health care costs associated with employees with diseases. Studies show that proper education of how to best deal with and live with chronic diseases can translate into lower health care costs versus those who are uneducated about to how best to life with and combat these health issues. Some of the common areas of disease management seen within worksite wellness programs include the following;

i.   **Diabetes**

ii. **Hypertension**

iii. **CHD**

iv. **Cancer**

c.   **Newsletters**

Healthy living newsletters are a great way to help promote the healthy lifestyle changes being highlighted in worksite wellness programs. This is also a great way to get the information out to family members of employees who are also covered by the health care plans provided by employers. Monthly newsletters are a great way to highlight many different issues as well as tips and tricks on how to live a healthier lifestyle. Workplaces that have a large group of medium to low risk individuals will benefit from a monthly or weekly newsletter.

d.   **Self-Study**

e.   **Screenings**

Another great way to promote health and health awareness is through providing employees with health screenings for major diseases and other likely health issues. These screenings are a way to allow your employees to get a glimpse of their current health and are also a launching point for discussions about how to improve health. Along with the screenings, provide educational material about how to combat these issues and improve their lifestyle. Providing incentives to getting screenings is a great way to increase the participation within these types of programs.

f. Seminars "Lunch and Learns"

Knowledge is power, and through seminars and presentations, workers will be able to better inform themselves about how to reduce their health care costs. A great way to do these seminars or presentations is by offering an incentive along with it. Provide a delicious and healthy lunch for employees who attend a health improvement seminar and it will increase participation.

g. Incentive Programs

Creating a series of incentives for employees who participate in worksite wellness programs is a great way to get the most amount of participation possible. Many employees may be reluctant to participate, and by creating a clear-cut incentive program, that number is likely to decrease.

Key Points

There are a number of different key points to keep in mind when it comes to pitching and creating a worksite wellness program inside a business or organization.

With these key points kept in mind the potential for the benefits of these programs are many.

Key Point - Worksite wellness programs benefit both the employee and employer in a number of different ways. While the employer may implement these programs in order to help them maintain costs and increase productivity, the benefits for employees are also very substantial.

Key Point - Worksite wellness programs help to lower costs of health care for both the employer and the employee. This is done through the increased education and collaborative effort of employee and employer participation in preventative measures and healthy choices.

Key Point - Worksite wellness programs improve employee morale, loyalty and productivity. Employees who see that their employer is putting in an extra effort to see that they are healthy and happy strive to work harder and perform better.

Key Point - Worksite wellness programs are shown to decrease employee absences, which in turn increases employee productivity.

Key Point - Employers are able to see a clear return on investment when worksite wellness programs are established and implemented in a beneficial manner. Positive wellness programs are shown to improve productivity, which in turn means higher revenue per employee towards company profits.

Summary

Worksite wellness programs can have a large impact on both the company and the individual employees. It is a way that a business can show the interest that they have for their employee's health while at the same time bettering their productivity and revenue. Worksite wellness programs have a number of benefits, all of them stemming from the goal of improving the overall health of their company's workforce. It is clear that a healthier workforce means a more productive workforce, and all of that can be achieved through a well put together and implemented worksite wellness program.

While the number crunching is beneficial in the amount of potential health care costs that can be saved, that is not the only visible benefit of a program such as this. Studies prove that an increased amount of education and a collaborative effort from health care providers and professionals in prevention education could have the potential to influence the larger health care industry. Workplace wellness programs are just one larger part of a step towards a healthier country that this nation so desperately needs.

As a RN, it is important to realize just how much of an impact can be made through programs such as this. You are already well equipped with the necessary education and through the necessary training and resources provided by L.I.T.E Therapeutics and HealthCoachNursingJobs.com; you have all of the necessary information to make this a part of your business.

RESOURCES AND TRAINING

The RN Health Coach Training Program found at www.HealthCoachNursingJobs.com provides potential worksite wellness coaches with all of the necessary information, training and resources they need to make this a part of their business. Any questions or advice needed for Registered Nurses to jump start this aspect of their RN Health Coaching business can be found here as well as through L.I.T.E. Therapeutics.

Post-Nursing Careers for RN's

Registered nurses gain valuable information, knowledge and experience throughout their careers as well as their education. The work that they perform as nurses is extensive and can be applied to a number of different industries. Registered nurses who have a reason or desire to step away from regular nursing jobs have a variety of other industries they are able to enter into. Being able to use the knowledge and experience they have gained within other industries can be very beneficial, to them as well as others.

The industries and areas that registered nurses are looking into for a career change, or simply a supplement to their nursing jobs, vary widely. Some of the many careers that are available to registered nurses include:

- Certified CPR & First Aid Training

- Medical Writing

- Insurance Industry Work

Training First Aid & CPR

There are a number of individuals who want to learn both first aid and CPR along with a number of businesses who require employees to be trained in one or both of these important areas. First aid and CPR training are important basics that can be beneficial for anyone to learn, especially those involved in physically active lifestyles. Many physically intensive industries require their employees to be trained in these areas as a way to help prevent, and properly deal with any workplace injuries.

There are a number of individuals and companies who need to be trained in first aid and CRP, and the certification these individuals gain commonly lasts between one and two years. This translates into the fact that first aid and CPR certification training is a need that will be ongoing. Jumping into this industry as a member of the medical community is a great way to share your knowledge as well as expand your career opportunities and income potential. Registered nurses are uniquely prepared and trained to instruct classes on first aid and CPR training.

RN's as First Aid and CPR Instructors

As a registered nurse, your experience and education make you a great candidate for an instructor in first aid and CPR training. Throughout your work experience, you have interacted with patients, are able to clearly explain medical circumstances and situations to others, and are dedicated to helping patients and clients. These are just a couple of the elements that make you, as a registered nurse, a great instructor for others wanting to learn and become certified within CPR and first aid.

Benefits of Being a CPR & First Aid Instructor

There are a number of benefits for registered nurses in becoming an instructor of first aid and CPR. Registered nurses have already gained a lot of experience and education within the medical field, which provides them with a great base for becoming qualified instructors. Many nurses are looking for a way to earn extra income, or take their knowledge and apply it to a different or supplemental career.

Nurses can see many benefits in stepping into a career as an instructor. Some of these benefits include:

• Community involvement

• Income and Career Potential

• Flexibility

Community Involvement

One of the benefits of becoming a CPR and First aid certified instructor is feeling the impact you are making in the community. Being able to be involved in the community and directly helping and affecting the ability of others to help is a large benefit of choosing this career path. It gives nurses the chance to connect with others in their community and truly impact their lives. The more people that are trained in first aid and CPR, the larger an impact your community will see

Income and Career Potential

CPR and first aid training is an area that will always be needed. Many businesses and schools require their employees to be trained in CPR and first aid as a precautionary and safety method. Some school teachers and daycare providers are required by law to maintain current CPR and first aid certification , which makes your potential client list endless.

Becoming a certified instructor allows you to be in control of your income and your career potential. The work that you put in will directly match the income and career that you get out. There is an almost unlimited demand for this knowledge, and it is in your hands to choose the type of career you can create out of it. For some it can serve as a great way to earn extra income on the side, and for others it can become their main career and source of income.

Flexibility

Many registered nurses who want to scale back their work schedule will find that certified instruction for CPR and first aid is a great way to take more control of your schedule. Being in charge of scheduling clients and training sessions is a great way to keep using the skills and knowledge that you have learned; however, at the same time being in more control. The flexibility that you can gain through creating a career as an instructor can be a great benefit for registered nurses wanting more control and flexibility of their work schedule.

Resources

Both the American Red Cross and the American Heart Association have a number of resources available for those wanting to get training and certification, as well as those wishing to become certified CPR teachers and trainers. The American Red Cross offers classes in CPR and First Aid training as well as other health related certifications such as swimming and lifeguard training. There are a number of opportunities for RN's to access through both the American Heart Association and the American red cross.

MEDICAL WRITING

The education and experience that registered nurses collect throughout the years of training and work is a solid base for a number of post-nursing careers. Medical writing is a great opportunity for nurses who are looking to step away from a highly physical nursing job and utilize their skills in other areas. It provides a great chance to supplement your income or in some cases, even replace your current position with a more flexible schedule.

What is Medical Writing?

Medical writing is a growing industry that focuses on the many different aspects involved in recording and communicating certain and often specific knowledge and ideas related to the medical field. Medical writing does not only cover the actual writing of these documents, but also includes a variety of writing and editing skills and positions. There are a number of different types and industries that use a variety of medical writing. This makes the potential for a medical writing job more available for those who are qualified.

Those who become involved with medical writing will produce a number of different documents related to the medical field. Documents can be created in order to describe and detail the results of a medical trial or be precise notes about a research project that is being conducted. Medical writers have a number of responsibilities, as it is their words that are putting the research into a readable format.

Medical writing takes a unique focus on the type of regulatory guidelines, medical journal guidelines and other formatting issues required to correctly produce a piece of writing. It is the job of the medical writer to turn the information gained into a readable piece of information that can be shared and understood clearly.

A medical writer's job can vary from industry to industry, and the type of writing that is needed can vary as well. Some medical writers focus on documenting trials and research studies from start to finish, while others may work specifically on the approval process for a drug or other medical device. Having an extensive knowledge of the medical field is a large benefit for those wishing to become a medical writer.

Industries that Need Medical Writers

Medical writing can span across many different industries, and your knowledge as a RN is a great start to a medical writing career. Nurses can apply their skills and knowledge as a medical writer in a number of industries including:

- Pharmaceuticals

- Research Facilities

- Drug and Medical Trials

- Government Agencies

- Non-profit Medical Sector

Qualifications of a Medical Writer

There are a number of basic qualifications that those wishing to become medical writers should take into account. Many of the qualifications are easily learned through experience and education by registered nurses and others who work closely within the medical or health care industry.

Some of the qualifications that medical writers should have, or be trained in, include:

- Knowledge of Medical Terms
- Clarity of Writing
- Knowledge of medical formatting rules and writing style guidelines
- Experience in the Medical Field

Knowledge of Medical Terms

Having a solid knowledge of a variety of medical terms is one of the most basic qualifications of a medical writer. Because the topics included within medical writing vary so greatly, it is necessary for any medical writer to have a grasp of both the English language as well as an extensive knowledge of medical terms and other medical jargon. This is necessary in order to properly understand and reiterate the medical information that you are provided with.

Throughout their education and experiences, registered nurses are required to learn a variety of different medical terminology and technical jargon. As their experience grows, so does their medical vocabulary, a skill that makes them uniquely qualified for a position in medical writing. Through the use of medical terms and knowledge of procedures written about and charted by nurses on a daily basis, their knowledge of medical terms becomes quite extensive.

Nurses spend a large portion of their jobs recording the patient's care and progress, and through this work, they get a handle on both common and less common medical terminology. Being able to both understand this terminology and write about it in a clear concise way, gives nurses a step up in the industry of medical writing.

Clarity of Writing

An important qualification of a good medical writer is to be able to present the information clearly and in a way that is easy for others to understand. Medical writers need to be concise with their writing and present the information in a straight forward and well written manner. Because the information is used for medical purposes, the importance of correctly explaining or detailing reports is a vital aspect of a medical writer.

Nurses are given the task of clearly writing out the activity of the patient, the history of what has been given to the patient, and keeping track of the progress and all medical related instances. One of the most important parts of a nurse's job is to be able to record all of this information, and record it in a way that is easy for others to understand. A registered nurses writing has been fine-tuned over years of producing charts, progress reports and notes about patients and their medical history.

Nurses are able to comprehend just how important it is to present the information in a manner that is clear and concise enough not to be misunderstood. It is their understanding of the negative consequences of having medical information misinterpreted that makes them diligent and highly quality medical writers.

Knowledge of Formatting and Style

Having knowledge of the writing style as well as formatting guidelines and rules within the medical industry is an important qualification of a medical writer. Many different formatting rules and writing styles are used within different aspects of the medical profession. It is important to have an understanding, and even better, to have extensive knowledge, of the many different styles and formatting rules and guidelines that are often used within medical writing.

As a registered nurse, your experience has allowed you access to a number of different styles. Many different clinics and hospitals vary in their formatting rules and guidelines. This has provided you with a unique chance to get a wide knowledge on these styles and medical writing gives you a chance to optimize your knowledge. While medical writing may not have initially been a direction in which you would go, it is your experience that has given you the set of skills you need.

Experience in the Medical Field

Having actual hands on experience within the medical field is a qualification that may not be necessary for a medical writer, but is definitely a clear benefit. Experience allows you as a writer to better understand and explain to another the medical topic you are writing about. It gives you a perspective that is necessary for effectively getting across the information you are preparing.

As a registered nurse, your experience within the medical field is extensive and varied. This provides you with a head start above others interested in medical writing. Because you have dealt with so many different patients, with different ailments and health issues, you have knowledge of many different health and medical related situations. This knowledge gives you a chance to better understand medical concepts as well as the information you are reporting on.

RN's as Medical Writers

Registered nurses have a number of qualities that make medical writing a great choice for a post-nursing or supplemental career. The experience that they have had within the health care industry makes them uniquely qualified to be a medical writer. Medical writers need to have a certain set of qualifications in order to be able to perform their job correctly, and many registered nurses already have these from the work they have done and experience they have.

Nurses who are considering a change in career do not have to let all of their work experience and the knowledge gained over the years go to waste. Instead, they should look at the skills that they have learned as transferrable to other aspects of the medical industries. Consider medical writing as an option for nurses looking to further their career in a less physical way. It is a chance to build on your knowledge and education and has a number of opportunities for any registered nurse looking for a change.

Benefits of Medical Writing for RNs

Medical writing has a number of benefits for registered nurses wanting to continue to use their education and experience but in a new and more flexible capacity. Medical writing jobs are available in many different areas and can be on-site work or in many cases, a work from home opportunity.

Many nurses, after working for years in a clinic or a hospital setting, want to find a new career with more flexibility. Medical writing gives nurses a chance to get more control when it comes to their career as well as their income and lifestyle. Some of the benefits of becoming a medical writer as a RN include the following:

- More Flexible Schedule
- Control of Income
- Control of Career Potential

Flexible Schedules

Medical writers have the unique opportunity to control just how much they work, and when they work. In many cases, medical writing can be done as a freelance position. What this means is that you take on as many clients as you want to or are able to. This allows you to control when you work and gives you a chance to plan work around an already busy schedule. Nurses who are also parents or wanting to become parents, find that the freelance aspect of medical writing is a great way to continue their career and start a family.

Control of Income

Along with the control of your working schedule, becoming a medical writer will also give you more control of your income. You are already equipped with many of the skills necessary to be successful, now the opportunity to make more income is completely up to how hard you want to work and the time you put in. The more experienced and efficient you become within the medical writing field will determine to how much you can charge. You are able to control the income you make, which gives you more control over your life.

Career Potential

The need for medical writing is endless and it will continue to be in high demand as long as the medical field is coming up with new technology and treatments. This provides any registered nurse with the unique opportunity to create their own career. There is unlimited potential when it comes to medical writing; it is up to you how much you put into it as well as how much you can get out. Developing a career in medical writing will take time, but it can be very rewarding financially.

Resources for Medical Writers

There are a number of companies and organizations in place to help those wishing to look further into the medical writing field. The American Medical Writers Association, www.amwa.org, as well as the Association of Health Care Journalists, www.healthjournalism.org, are great sources for additional information, training and job opportunities.

In addition, there have been a number of books published about the details of the medical writing industry. Author Cynthia Saver published the "Anatomy of Writing for Publication for Nurses," which is a helpful resource for RN's looking into the medical writing field. Another book that looks into succeeding within the medical writing field is "The Writers Workbook: Health Professionals Guide to getting Published," written by Shirley H. Fondiller.

INSURANCE INDUSTRY

There are a number of opportunities for registered nurses looking for a career change within the insurance industry. Health insurance companies are often looking for nurses who are able to use their knowledge and experience to help in a variety of areas from performing physicals for potential members to reading and reviewing medical charts. If you are a registered nurse looking for a change in pace and careers, the health insurance industry may have an opportunity for you. Some of the jobs that registered nurses can be qualified for or trained for within health insurance companies include:

- Case Managers

- Clinical Chart Review

- Conducting Entry Physicals

- Claim Review

Case Managers

Registered nurses are very capable of handling a number of different patient's charts and information at the same time, and it is this that helps them to become more qualified to work as a case manager within an insurance company. Insurance companies often hire bedside RN's as case managers because of their ability to multi task as well as the experience that they have dealing with patients and doctors on a day to day basis. This experience gives nurses the unique qualifications to make highly capable and effective case managers.

Case managers within a health insurance company are responsible for a number of different aspects involved in the overall care of the member and patient. Some of the responsibilities include contacting the patient and insuring they are informed about their medications, remaining in contact with their doctors, and receiving any necessary treatments.

It is this aspect of patient care that carries over from a registered nurses experiences and knowledge that makes them qualified for this type of position.

Clinical Chart Review

A large part of a bedside nurses responsibilities is recording and properly charting a patient's progress and treatment. Throughout the years, a registered nurse will have gone over and through a number of patient charts making them uniquely qualified to be able to read and understand what a chart is saying. This is a quality that can be used within the health insurance industry when it comes to the reviewing of clinical charts.

Registered nurses are well qualified for the position within an insurance company that focuses on clinical chart review. They are able to look at a chart and determine if the necessary care was provided or if the care provided was above what was necessitated by the patients' health status.

It is very detailed oriented work, something that as a registered nurse, you have had experience with. While this may not be the best fit for all nurses, it is an area that nurses can step into without further training.

Conducting Physicals

Almost every health insurance company requires their applicants to agree to a physical evaluation before accepting their application and providing them with a quote for the cost of coverage. Many of these insurance companies will turn to registered nurses as a way to execute these physicals in a way that is non-biased and is considered accurate.

Insurance companies often hire a number of nurses who work from home and travel to the members home or business to perform the simple evaluations. These nurses are often compensated on a per visit structure. This means that the more clients they see and evaluate, the more their income will be. This is a great source of extra income and gives you the chance to be flexible about your schedule and when, or how often, you work.

Benefits of Working with Insurance Companies

After serving as a bedside registered nurse for a number of years, many of these individuals want a change of scenery or more control over their work schedule. Working with a health insurance company in a variety of capacities provides you with the opportunity to use the skills that you have gained and the education you have relied on in a different application. There are so many different chances and work opportunities for registered nurses within the insurance industry that you are able to find one that suits you.

If you want to continue to work closely with patients and influence a person's life on an everyday basis, working as a registered nurse case manager is a way to continue to do that. It is a job that allows you to have much more control and flexibility than a traditional bedside nursing job would. You have the chance to choose when you work, where you work and how often you work. Nursing jobs within the insurance industry gives registered nurses many chances including:

- Making Use of Your Skills
- Job Flexibility
- Work from Home Opportunities

Nurses who want to change careers but not abandon the work and education they have put into their nursing jobs will find a number of opportunities within the insurance industry. You are uniquely able to continue to take advantage of everything that you have learned and experienced and apply it to a new and different set of job requirements. This will not only expand your knowledge, but also make you more capable of changing paths in the future.

Stepping away from bedside nursing not only gives you more opportunities, but also allows you to have more flexibility. After working strange hours and long shifts, using your knowledge within the insurance industry gives you a chance to regain more normal working hours. You are able to better create the life you want and be more flexible with how you structure you working schedule.

Many of the jobs offered within the insurance industry for registered nurses are available in a work from home capacity. This is a great option for those who want to spend more time at home or get away from the stressful hospital situations. Working from home and earning the same amount of money is a goal that many registered nurses will want to achieve.

Resources for Insurance Industry

The health insurance provider Aetna, www.aetna.com, has a number of resources and opportunities for registered nurses looking to join the insurance industry. In addition, the company McKesson, www.mckesson.com, provides helpful information as well as opportunities.

Key Points

There are a number of key points to remember from the information we discussed in this chapter.

Key Point - Registered nurses are uniquely qualified to transfer the skills they have learned to a variety of other industries and job opportunities.

Key Point - Becoming a certified CPR and first aid trainer is a great way to increase your income or substitute your current bedside nursing job with flexibility and income potential.

Key Point - Medical writing is an industry that registered nurses can take advantage of and earn supplementary income. It can provide work flexibility and unlimited income potential with the knowledge RN's already contain.

Key Point - The insurance industry is in need of qualified registered nurses to assist them in a number of different capacities.

Key Point - The work and experience that RN's have make them qualified to perform chart reviews, become case managers, or become traveling nurses for insurance company physicals.

Summary

Many individuals who have been registered nurses in the traditional capacity are ready for a career change after years of grueling schedules and work. At the same time, they do not want to throw away the work and experience they have gained over the years. This work and experience makes them qualified to transfer the knowledge to other industries and job potentials.

Becoming certified in CPR and first aid, as well as starting a career within the insurance industry or as a medical writer are all different paths a registered nurse looking for a career change can go down. It is important to take into account the type of area you want to go into. Each of the ones discussed in this chapter can provide you with job flexibility as well as a high amount of income potential. It is important to find a new career that fits your goals and desires as a RN and as an individual.

SPEAKING/SEMINARS

Nurse Experts as Speakers and Seminar Leaders

Speaking and Seminars

Every year there are hundreds upon hundreds of health care related seminars, conferences, conventions, expos and symposiums that are held all across the country. At each of these meetings, there are a number of different speakers and experts featured to discuss a variety of topics and issues within the health care industry.

The background of speakers and seminar leaders can vary greatly from doctors and nursing experts to administrators and researchers. There are a number of opportunities for field and topic experts to appear as a featured speaker at many types of meetings and conferences.

Within a single seminar, there are a number of different speeches and presentations made by various experts. As a registered nurse, these conventions and meetings provide you with a great opportunity to make the best out of the knowledge and experience that you already have within the health care industry. With your direct experience within the health care and nursing industries, you are able to provide significant insight which can be helpful to a number of people.

As technology advances so does the reach, span and influence of any type of seminar or meeting. In many cases, the technology of the internet has provided the opportunity to create your own virtual meetings, which will create a limitless chance of speaking opportunity and income.

Registered Nurses as Seminar Leaders

As a registered nurse, you are uniquely qualified to take advantage of the opportunities available to take part in a number of different types of seminars as a speaker. It is both your education as well as work experience that has prepared you with the knowledge necessary to be a successful and influential speaker. Registered nurses have a number of opportunities to increase their income through participating in conventions and other guest-speaking. There are an infinite number of opportunities to take advantage of when it comes to speaking as a nurse expert. It is this that allows nurse experts to be able to control the amount of money that they earn.

Benefits of Speaking

There are a number of different benefits to becoming a guest expert nurse speaker. Taking advantage of the chances to share your knowledge and experience with others is a great way to take control of your working schedule. It also provides you with an influential and easy way to supplement your income as well as share your experience. Many nurses who are looking for career options that do not involve long hours and have large income potential have found that speaking is a great and readily available option.

About the Speaking Industry

The speaking industry has played an important role in the business and development for a number of different industries. It allows fellow industry members the opportunity to connect and discuss current and important issues and topics in a variety of ways.

Conferences, meetings and presentations are a great way to disseminate important information as it allows you to directly impact those who are participating in those industries. These are just a few of the many positive aspects of the speaking industry that will enable it to continue to have a strong and constant presence across many fields of study.

As the country becomes more technologically involved, so does the speaking industry. This can be seen in the number of recorded presentations, seminars and speeches that are available for purchase in a number of different subject areas. In fact, many experts will continually put on virtual meetings as a way to provide information and increase their income potential.

There are a number of available opportunities within the speaking industry for a nurse expert. Because knowledge is so greatly desired, the hard part is not finding those who want to learn, but in creating a strategy to attract and capture their attention. With the right training, education and resources, registered nurses would be able to greatly increase their income or even possible replace their old career.

How you as a RN can benefit from the speaking industry

Registered nurses have a number of different ways that they can take advantage of the speaking industry through the sharing of knowledge and experience. Registered nurses are well prepared for interaction, explaining the consequences and outcomes of certain diseases, treatments and care as well as being well educated. Becoming a speaker allows registered nurses to optimize on the education they have already earned and share it in a new way to a number of people who will greatly benefit from the information.

One great benefit for nurses is knowing that they are still having a large impact on the health of individuals. A great RN speaker is not only informative but enjoys sharing the experiences they have had and the knowledge that has been gained through these experiences.

Speech and Seminar Topics for Nurses

There are a number of different topics and issues that registered nurses are qualified to speak on and would provide a unique view and information. With additional education and training, the range of topics that can be covered by nurse experts are almost unlimited.

Some nurses will choose to pay particular attention to a certain type of issue such as weight loss and will learn extensively about that topic. In the other case, some nurses decide to gain a general knowledge that spans over a number of different topics to be able to widen the types of conferences or seminars in which they will be able to take part.

Topics can vary greatly on subject matter and may change over time as health care issues and trends change with the society that we currently live in. Some of the common topics for speeches and seminars led by nurses include the following:

• Weight Loss

  Our country has made it clear that there is currently a very large problem with obesity and weight related health issues. It is estimated that over 2 billion people will be considered overweight across the globe by 2013 according to the World Health Organization. This is just one piece of evidence that points out how much of a need there is to have well educated speakers that can impact the knowledge such issues.

This is going to be an important issue stepping forward into the future, as there are a number of different health related diseases that stem from obesity. It is important to share the knowledge of the potential risks of being overweight and the problems it can cause in the future.

- Smoking Cessation

  Smoking is still problematic across our nation and it affects millions of people who are unable to get away from its addictive properties. Nurse experts who are knowledgeable about the best ways to quit smoking will be able to find opportunities to share their knowledge in a number of speaking situations. There is also a great need for experts to share and spread the consequences of smoking to the younger generation as a means of prevention. There are many opportunities to be a speaker at schools across the country as a nurse expert on this topic as well as others.

- Disease Management

  Learning how to best manage a number of common diseases is a very important topic when it comes to health care provided by nurses as well as by family members and support systems. Acquiring expertise on how to best deal with common chronic illnesses such as high blood pressure and diabetes, will enable you to become part of a number of health care related conferences and seminars.

- Worksite Wellness

  Worksite wellness is an aspect of business-provided health care that has had large emphasis placed on it in recent years. Worksite wellness includes any number of campaigns to promote overall health among workers. One of the aspects of many different worksite wellness plans is the inclusion of guest speakers who would provide information on common workplace and health issues.

- Patient Care

  Patient care is an aspect of health care that will always be important and requires a certain amount of attention and education in order to improve. As a registered nurse, you are already well versed in what is required in positive and beneficial patient care and you are able to share your experience and knowledge with others who are in the same situations.

- Healthy Living

  There are a number of different types of speaking opportunities when it comes to topics surrounding healthy living. It is an important part of everyday life and many people constantly try to strive towards leading a more healthy life, but they may not know exactly how to achieve it.

  As a nurse, you are well equipped with the knowledge needed to help others improve the quality of their health and lifestyle. With further education and training, you can create a number of opportunities to take advantage of sharing this knowledge and information with others who are eager to listen and learn about this topic.

- Career Development

  As a nurse expert, backed with training and education, you are able to help others start off in their nursing career. There are a number of different seminars based on establishing yourself as a nurse, and even going beyond normal nursing careers and reaching for more. This is a topic that will always be present and can be utilized by any nurse experts looking to further their education and share their experiences and success strategies with others.

- Motivational Speaking

  Motivational speaking is a type of presentation or speech that will continue to dominate the conference and convention industry. There is always a point in everyone's life when they need a little extra boost or a kick in the rear to get where they are going and achieving what they are capable of. This is where the realm of motivational speaking has such a large impact. As a nurse expert, your experience gives you a good amount of perspective on perseverance in the face of hardships as well as hard work and determination.

  These are just a sample of common topics that are discussed, however any number of topics can be spoken about by nurses and nurse experts. Finding a topic that interests you as a person and has an impact on you is a great way to create an experience for your audience that moves them to action.

- Developing Speaking expertise

  There are a number of different ways to develop speaker expertise from continued education, as well as training. There is an art to being able to give a speech and have those who are listening be influenced enough to take action on the topic on which you are speaking. While as a nurse expert you already have the knowledge required to become a speaker, it is important to spend time on improving your speaking expertise as well as learning more about the topic you are discussing.

There are a number of programs offered by companies that are geared at preparing educated individuals on how to best take advantage of a speaking career. Through these companies and their resources and tools, you will be able to better create a presentation that has a large impact and grabs attention.

Resources for Speakers

There are a number of different programs and resources that are available to help nurse experts themselves develop as better speakers. It is programs such as these that will be able to provide nurses with the knowledge and training to improve their speaking as well as the delivery and effectiveness of a presentation. Some of the well-known resources for those looking into a speaking career include the following:

- Toastmasters Organization

  The Toastmasters Organization is a group that is dedicated to improving your speaking ability. This is a great tool for nurses with the education and experience to speak on, but are looking for more guidance about how to deliver these speeches.

- Seminar Education Companies

  Getting involved with seminar education companies is a good way to get more training and expertise. Working alongside companies such as Fred Pryor Career Track will give you extra preparation in starting a speaking career. This company and their supporting website, www.pryor.com, has a number of resources to help you develop yourself as a speaker and seminar leader.

- National Speakers Association

  The National Speakers Association provides experts who wish to create a business out of their knowledge with a number of different aspects involved in stepping into the speaking industry. It is an association made up of a number of experts ranging from a number of different industries all with the goal of creating a business out of presenting their knowledge to others. Members benefit from others knowledge and the ability to learn and grow in an educational community.

- TheNurseExpert.com

  The Nurse Expert provides information that is directly relatable to nurses wishing to further the use of their education and training by embarking on the journey into the speaking industry. The Nurse Expert provides both an online course available on their website as well as a series of books, The Nurse Expert Book Series. The volume 3 of the Nurse Expert Book series provides a number of details when it comes to speech delivery.

This site offers a number of different ways that nurses can optimize on this opportunity and present the best speech possible. Some of the aspects that are covered by The Nurse Expert include that of creating high quality speeches and learning how to best network and create speech giving opportunities for yourself.

Qualifications of a Good Speaker

There are a number of different factors that influence the quality and effectiveness of a speaker and many speakers have different qualities. When it comes to starting out as a speaker it is important to keep in mind the measures by which one is judge and looked at by others listening and watching you. Some of the main qualifications include the following aspects of speaking:

- Being Eloquent

  One of the most obvious aspects of a successful speaking career is that of being able to properly express yourself. Being able to clearly demonstrate the point you are trying to make through simple and understandable words is an important trait for a successful speaker to have. Understanding how the art of speech impacts the effectiveness of a presentation is something that needs to be mastered in order to succeed in this type of industry. It allows you to present a powerful seminar or speech that will impact those watching and listening.

- Displaying Expertise

  Everything is good and well when it is said by someone; however, the impact is far less if that person does not have the expertise to back up their claims. Claims made by an uninformed individual will not carry the same amount of weight as claims made by an expert in the field. Their knowledge and skill set are greater and therefore are more easily relied upon by others both within and outside of their industry.

- Purpose and Determination

    In order to have a successful career as a speaker, it is important that you are determined and hardworking. It is not something that will develop overnight, but rather takes a certain amount of effort in order to get it off the ground. Showing that you have that purpose and determination is what makes you a great potential speaker as a nurse expert.

- Who you are as a person

    It is important that you represent and present yourself in a way that coincides with the work you are trying to do as a speaker. This touches on all of the areas of importance, and should not be forgotten. Reputation and the integrity of your character are all important parts of creating a successful speaking career.

Potential Income for Keynote Speakers

There is a large amount of income potential when it comes to becoming a keynote speaker. When you are extremely knowledgeable in a certain subject area, your knowledge is well paid for and compensated. Keynote speakers are able to decide just how much they want to make and can schedule their appearances around the income goal.

The amount a normal keynote speaker would charge to appear at a convention or to present a speech varies greatly on the topic, length of presentation and history of the individual's past work and experience. The more credentials and experience that you create for yourself, the more you will be able to charge for your time, and the more financial freedom you will establish.

One of the main factors in cost and payment for speakers is how long the function is. In some cases, it may only be an hour, and in others, it may last a full day or even over a weekend. In many cases, speakers who are just starting out will start with shorter presentations until they build up a reputation and work history. In many cases entry level speakers with expertise and desired knowledge can make upwards of $2,500-$4000 when it comes to speaking for just over one hour.

As you begin to create more of a reputation around your speaking and the presentations you show, you will be able to increase this number. Celebrity motivational speakers for example are known to make over $15,000 for every appearance that they make, which is usually on the shorter side. While this money may not be realistic to start off with, it is good to know that it is possible to earn a large amount of extra income.

For nurses who enter into this field with determination and drive, they will be better equipped and able to create the type of lifestyle they want with this type of career. The amount of income that can be made is entirely up to you and how much you are willing to and want to put into the equation. The more time spent with education and additional training, the more you will be considered an expert or qualified to talk about the topic. This will translate directly to the amount of money you are usually paid for these appearances.

This opportunity also leaves the flexibility of working for yourself on the table. You are able to decide how many or how little appearances and speeches you will make. If you are trying to create a full time job out of professionally speaking, you have the option to work harder and create a larger association with other speakers and meeting companies.

Additional Revenue from Seminars

Once you have begun to establish yourself as a qualified and expert speaker on a topic, it is easy to create even more revenue with seminars and conferences. As your expertise grows and you continue to educate yourself, you will be able to optimize on this through the use of merchandise. This could be recordings of presentations, or books written by you about the topic you are speaking in.

Some other ways of creating extra revenue from seminars is by selling merchandise. Some examples of extra revenue tools include selling books, audio programs or DVDs that focus on the topic that you are speaking about.

By selling extra merchandise related to your expertise throughout these presentations, you will see a number of benefits. First and most clearly, you will see the addition of revenue from seminars that do not come from admissions or the actual speech. In addition, you will be able to spread the word about who you are and what your focus is through the use of multimedia for sale to your viewers.

Benefits of Meeting Groups

There are a number of different associations that are available to join and that you would benefit from. Some of these are free and others are fee based; however, the fees are generally minimal and worth the amount paid. Some of the most common associations within the speaking industry are that of meeting groups.

Meeting groups are organizations that are focused on providing specific meetings for a group from an industry or company. These meeting groups are in charge of finding speakers for conferences, expos and conventions of all different sorts. As a nurse expert trying to get into this type of industry, it is a good idea to make as many possible connections as you can.

One of the simple ways to make connections that will last is through joining a meeting group such as the one found at   www.mpiweb.org, the Meeting Planners International.

This group in particular provides a number of different resources for both those looking to host meetings as well as those looking to be included as a speaker or seminar leader for these meetings. There are also many online webinars that are made available through these websites that will help to improve a speaker's effectiveness.

Professional Seminar Providers

Another way to take advantage of the resources offered within the field of speaking is through the association with seminar providing companies. Many companies have been created to plan and execute educational seminars for a number of different topics as well as a number of different industries. As an entry level speaker, it is important to realize the impact that these types of organizations could have on your effect and rate of growth.

There are a number of different types of connections that can be made when using these programs. While part of the benefits can be found in the resources and education available, another important aspect to look at is the community that you are joining. Being able to learn from and feed off of other successful speakers is a great way to learn how to best accomplish making this into a career that can last and provide for you.

Using Associations as Clients and Resources

Topic specific associations can be a great resource in a number of different capacities. Nurse experts can take advantage of topic specific associations by considering them as potential clients. For example, nurses who are beginning a speaking career focused on healthy living may consider approaching an association whose goal is to promote healthy living. This is a great way to get access to your target audience all in one place, and it gives you the opportunity to establish a relationship with an association that will continue to need your services over a long period of time.

The other way that topic specific associations can be used as a resource is by giving you more insight into the audience you are trying to target. By becoming a part of and getting active in a specific association, you are able to learn more about your audience and how best to approach and relate to them throughout your speaking career.

Key Points

We have talked about a number of different topics that can come up when trying to create a successful speaking career, as well as the number of benefits these careers can have on a registered nurse.

Key Point - There are countless opportunities for registered nurses to jump into the speaking industry because of their education and experience.

Key Point - The income potential that a keynote speaker can reach is dependent on their drive and determination, as well as how much and often they want to work.

Key Point - The more experience you gain, along with the training and education you take advantage of, is directly relatable to the amount that you will be compensated for as a speaker.

Key Point - As a speaker, it is important to be eloquent, knowledgeable, true to yourself, and confident.

Key Point - Utilizing groups and associations such as meeting planners and seminar providers is a great way to become established as a speaker, as well as gain experience and job history speaking on certain topics.

Key Point - Nurse expert speakers can become successful by focusing mainly on one specific topic or sub topic, but they can also have success by gaining knowledge over a number of different topics. This helps to expand the type of speaking that you will be assigned or asked to present.

Key Point - There are a number of resources that are available that will help to make you a better speaker. Some of these include the tools and resources at thenurseexpert.com

Summary

The field of speaking is one that is continuing to grow and expand. The expertise of others who are more knowledgeable is always valued by those eager to learn and experience more things. It is important to know that as a nurse expert, you are able to provide this type of knowledge and expertise you have gained through experience.

There is a large amount of untapped income potential within the speaking industry, and when your knowledge and experience is paired with determination and hard work, you will be able to fully grasp the opportunity. This type of work puts you in charge of your schedule, what you learn and discover as well as what kind of lives you affect through your speaking.

Nurse experts often find that hired speaking is a great way to influence many people and share knowledge that could change lives. It is important to remember that being properly trained and ready to speak is an important part of being successful in this field. It is important to use the tools and resources made available to you.

HOLISTIC NURSING

Concept of Holistic Nursing

"The world is put back by the death of everyone who has to sacrifice the development of his or her peculiar gifts to conventionality." This quotation by Florence Nightingale, considered one of the very first holistic nurses, captures the essence of holistic nursing. Her brave willingness to develop gifts and skills that defied convention was the driving force behind the successful English nurse, writer and statistician. Holistic nursing is a specialty area that, to this day, focuses on Ms. Nightingale's philosophy of providing a totality of treatment, that is, healing based on treatment of the mind, body, emotions and spirit-the whole person.

While holistic therapies were an unconventional idea in her day, the concept of holistic nursing is a widely adopted approach to healing around the world today. In the above quote, Ms. Nightingale is lamenting the loss potential resulting from those who live with fear of thinking "outside of the box," so to speak. Does Florence Nightingale's quotation strike a familiar chord in your own nursing career goals? Are you unwilling to sacrifice your unique nursing gifts for the sake of following convention? If not, let us introduce you to the interesting and rewarding career of holistic nursing.

Today, holistic nurses are recognized as a focused nursing practice area. Traditionally, Western medicine approached healing by treating symptoms as they arose. The holistic approach to medicine also addresses symptoms but primarily focuses on treatment of the entire human being, inside and out. It is not so much of a practice as a viewpoint and philosophy that seeks to address and heal issues involving the life experience of the total person, including environment and social behaviors.

The popularity of holistic nursing increased as more people became willing to try alternative options for their health treatment. With the constant change in traditional medical treatment, many medical practitioners in the West are embracing this approach to treatment. For example, you are most likely aware of the work done by National Institutes of Health (NIH), the medical research agency of the United States. However, did you know that this U.S. Department of Health & Human Services agency regularly conducts research and clinical trials to broaden the spectrum of available holistic therapies? Indeed, holistic nursing is becoming a more accepted practice, even in the "official" medical practice arena.

Holistic nursing is not meant to replace or to undermine conventional medical treatment. However, it is a means for patients to receive complementary treatment that results in the most successful healing that is possible. One unique feature of holistic nursing is that it focuses on digging deep into illness, past the symptoms, until a root cause is uncovered. The American Holistic Nurses' Association defines it as a nursing practice with the goal of healing the whole person.

Fundamentals Uses of Holistic Medicine

Globally, millions of people use holistic medicine to:

- Heal chronic and grave illness
- Prevent physical and emotional illness and disease

- Treat mental disorders

- Achieve and maintain healthy weight

- Treat acute symptoms of illness

- Increase energy and maintain overall good health

As a holistic nurse, you play a key role in the success of those you treat.

Holistic Nursing Duties

Included among the duties that holistic nurses perform is the ability to incorporate several health practices when caring for patients. As a holistic nurse, your goal should be to provide not just physical well being of your patient, but to treat the mental, spiritual and emotional health of the individual. This is accomplished by deciding upon treatments based upon the overall physical health along with respecting the spiritual beliefs of the individual.

The multi-faceted aspect of holistic nursing utilizes treatment that includes non-traditional methods. Depending upon the treatment plan for the individual patient, some typical duties of a holistic nurse may include the following:

- Applying massage therapy treatments

- Drafting appropriate nutritional plans

- Spiritual support and exercises such as prayer

- Suggesting and selecting healing music

- Physical activities such as dance and exercise

- Traditional treatment as appropriate

As a holistic nurse, it is important for you to remember that a diagnosis serves to identify not just potential problems in the patient, but their strengths as well. The foremost goal for their spiritual care is to mobilize their own spiritual resources; not attempt to convert them to a particular viewpoint. In response to needs that are expressed, interventions should be made only by the patient's permission or request. Remember, the spiritual assessment should be carefully made and based upon your respect and awareness of the cultural, social and spiritual preference of the patient. Never hesitate to recognize your own limitations and request assistance if needed.

Holistic nursing incorporates complementary and alternative healing modalities into clinical practice (CAM). It is important for you to get a full understanding of these modalities in order to treat patients effectively. The categories of these modalities are outlined by the National Center for Complementary and Alternative Medicine as follows:

Mind and Body Medicine. This modality includes the utilization of methods such as art and color therapy, music therapy, and yoga in patient treatment. It also includes counseling and psychotherapy treatments and other therapies such as hypnotherapy and meditation, stress management and neuro-linguistic programming (NLP).

Biologically based practices. This includes practices such as herbal therapy and nutritional counseling. Also included in this category is biofeedback, which utilizes electronic monitoring of automatic body functions, such as heart rate and blood pressure, to train patients to gain voluntary control of the same function.

Hydrotherapy is another biologically based practice, which uses water and exercise to provide pain relief and treat illness.

Whole medical systems. These include homeopathy, or the treatment of illness with natural substances that would cause disease in a healthy person; or osteopathy, which is medical treatment involving manipulation of the musculoskeletal system.

Body based practices. These include acupuncture, acupressure and other such treatments. Acupuncture is a treatment originating with traditional Chinese medicine that treats pain by inserting needles into specific areas of the body. Acupressure, a derivative of acupuncture, is the application of physical pressure to the acupuncture points throughout the body. Physical therapies, chiropractic medicine and aromatherapy treatments are included in this category.

Energy medicine. Treatment includes many Eastern healing methods such as Chi Kung and the administration of alternative therapies such as Reiki and Reflexology. Energy medicine may require the holistic nurse to administer magnetic therapy and spiritual treatment such as prayer or meditation.

The modalities described above can also be distinguished by the three areas that they treat. Modalities that treat the body include biofeedback and therapeutic massage. Those that relieve the mind are imagery, humor, meditation and the like. In addition, the soul is comforted with prayer and other spiritual exercise.

Holistic nursing offers incredibly flexible and endless options for treatment. It is a rewarding, challenging and interesting career for people like you who desire to use their skills, gifts and talents to promote wholeness and health.

Protection of the client. In addition to providing the best holistic care possible, as a nurse you have a duty to protect the patient from danger. In a clinical setting, it is the duty of the holistic nurse to report any activities, medical or otherwise, that pose a danger to the patient.

Nursing Plan. As you are well aware, nurses must be sure to develop plans for nursing care. The purpose of the nursing care plan includes diagnosis and goal setting to identify needs. Determining interventions and their implantation is also included. Never forget the importance of the nursing care plan and the characteristics of an effective plan. In review, the most important thing is that the plan is thorough. The exact format will vary greatly depending on the setting. There are, however, basic sections you should remember that should be incorporated into the plan which include:

- The objective as well as subjective information about the patient. This comprehensive assessment will document the age, symptoms and medical history.

- List all problems that may affect treatment. Include medical conditions, family problems, nutritional issues, etc.

- Planning and treatment will detail specific goals for patient care. The instructions in this section should be able to be followed by any member of a nursing staff.

- The evaluation report includes tests that need to be performed and how the patient responds to treatment.

- Remember to update the care plan as the patient recovers. Don't neglect to record an updated version of the points as discussed above.

- Do not hesitate to get assistance with how to prepare a nursing plan. Nursing plan templates and information are widely available.

Ethics

Nursing care is not restricted by race, nationality, sex or sexual preference, age or social status. As professional caregivers, nurses must understand the diverse cultural backgrounds of patients and their families in order to utilize interventions appropriate with the various cultures. It is the fundamental responsibility of a nurse to promote and facilitate health and healing and to eliminate suffering to the best extent possible.

It is the nurse's responsibility to be a model of health care by striving to achieve balance and harmony in his or her own life. The patient is the nurse's most important responsibility. The patient should therefore be viewed as whole and should be respected. Patients should be assured that their information is held in complete confidence; a nurse should be diligent in using professional judgment when disclosure is absolutely necessary.

A holistic nurse is required to understand and maintain relationships with other health professionals. If applicable, the holistic nurse should be able to utilize research findings in the course of directing practice. They support holistically oriented nursing theories and practices. It is the responsibility of the nurse to create an environment of nurturing, harmony and peace to promote healing. Holistic nurses take into consideration the relation of the health in the ecosystem to the need that all people have for safety, health and peace.

Qualifications

If you are interested in this field of medicine, either to work for someone else or to open your own practice, it is important to know what is expected in order to succeed in this career.

The specialty practice of holistic nursing is dependent upon the education, expertise and intuition of practicing nurses. These characteristics are what guide the nurses to become so called "instruments" of healing. Holistic nurses are considered partners with the patients in their care. They must recognize and accept the human being in totality in order to provide effective therapy for patients.

A professional holistic nurse has also mastered the ability to integrate responsibility, self care, reflection and spirituality into his or her own life, which is the path to awareness of how to successfully treat the patient holistically.

However, holistic nurses are specially trained to respect and honor every person's health beliefs and values. The nurse must at all times strike a harmonious balance between honoring a patient's experiences while facilitating healing; which is one of the ways in which your "particular" and "unique" gifts can be utilized in holistic nursing.

A holistic or any other nurse should have a caring nature with the ability to communicate by their actions that they care for their patients. They should be empathetic to people who are frightened or in pain. All nurses must be stable emotionally since there are many emotional ups and downs on any working day. If these are your natural characteristics, your job will be very rewarding.

Attention to detail is extremely important for every nurse for duties such as charting treatments and administering treatments or medication. Since each day is different, nurses must be flexible and able to adapt quickly to a variety of circumstances. If you are a quick thinker with great instincts and communication skills, you will most likely have an awesome career in holistic nursing.

Education

To become a holistic nurse, you must be a qualified registered nurse with a bachelor's degree and certification in holistic nursing. Although most holistic nurses hold bachelor's degrees in nursing, it is not mandatory to hold the degree in this field. It is recommended, however, since pursuing a nursing degree allows students to work with licensed medical professionals and to explore various hospital settings and patients in their clinical studies.

In order to qualify, registered nurses are required to successfully finish a healing arts program in order to be certified. Many higher learning institutions offer special programs that prepare nurses for certification. Upon completion of these programs, nurses are equipped with the training and education and the needed understanding of the concept behind holistic nursing. It is quite common to get complementary practice certification in addition to general holistic nursing.

The Holistic Nurse Certification (HNC) is a very popular national certification awarded by the American Holistic Nurses' Certification Corporation (AHNCC). Certification through AHNCC is recognized throughout this industry to represent that a nurse has a commitment to holistic nursing as well as advanced holistic nursing practice skills.

The program offers three distinct certification programs for nurses without degrees, nurses with bachelor's degrees and advanced holistic nursing certification. All information regarding the certification process, including credentials, fees and eligibility criteria, are detailed on the AHNCC website. But where are these well qualified, caring and skilled holistic nurses employed?

Employment

Holistic nurses work in any nursing field such as oncology, surgery or pediatrics. They are employed in hospitals, holistic clinics, and hospitals and acupuncture offices. Wellness centers, fitness programs, doctors' offices, home health care businesses also employ holistic nurses. Holistic nurses hold positions as holistic treatment nurses, teachers (both online and in person), researchers and many other jobs.

Private Nursing Practice

An increasingly common decision that nurses such as you have made is to maintain their own holistic nursing practice. Imagine the endless possibilities that open for a well qualified holistic nurse in private practice. You can practice holistic nursing using several therapies and healing techniques. You have the opportunity to experience the rewards and challenges of utilizing your skills to help others. A private nursing practice gives you the freedom to set your own hours and change locations if desired.

As with any new venture, the importance of planning cannot be stressed enough. Don't be shy about digging deep within and asking the hard questions. Develop your own plan that starts with identifying your unique personal and professional vision. This means taking some time alone and giving careful thought to the important goals you have for your life.

Visualize your ideal work life with regard to time and vacation flexibility, whether you desire to work alone or with others, support system and other issues. Remember, your personal life must be in line with your professional vision. Otherwise, the chances of achieving your goal are greatly diminished. Therefore, do not rush through this important step in the process.

Equally important to the process is taking care of the setting up of the business. This includes being well informed about applicable business license you will need as well as state Board certification and licensure.

Setting up your business also includes making decisions about the location for your business. Most beginning entrepreneurs that need to save money on overhead look into alternative options for office space. Some holistic nurses save expenses by working from home. Naturally, this would only work if you plan to specialize in providing services that can be performed from home. Consultation, online teaching, nursing recruitment and research are services that may be ideal for a home based business. If you need office space for your practice, consider sharing office space (and expenses) with another professional until your business grows.

You will need to open a bank account for your business and begin having marketing materials such as business cards printed. Financial funding, bookkeeping, taxes and insurance are other important matters that must be taken care of. Although the tasks may seem daunting, you can achieve your goal with patience and planning.

Experienced holistic nurses with their own practices offer several tips for nurses new to the industry including:

- Always remain clear about the scope of your practice. A review of the Nurse Practice Act is imperative in order for you to know for sure that you have the legal right to perform duties plan to do as a holistic nurse. Your practice must fit within both the definition and the scope of practice for a registered nurse in your state or you might be violating the law. Be sure to check the definition of your particular state, as they are different in each state.

- The National Council of State Boards of Nursing website lists contact information for every state ; be sure to consult this and your own state Board administrative rules.

- Start early building a support base. This includes family and friends who will provide support and advice, colleagues and other medical professionals. Join as many professional organizations as possible. These resources will be valuable for networking conferences, advice, emotional support and other benefits of membership.

- One of the best ways to improve your chances of success is to keep your goals within reason. Take small steps that you will most likely easily complete; this will build your confidence and experience. Don't sabotage your own success by planning unrealistic goals.

- The nursing industry is rightly well regulated and governed with strict sanctions for non-compliance. Don't take chances with your practice. Know the laws in your state regarding the practice of holistic nursing. In addition, make sure you are aware of the legalities related to any business matters such as partnerships or other contracts. If necessary, hire an attorney to look at any legal paperwork that you are unsure of.

Whether in a clinical setting, home environment or private practice, it is the full responsibility of the nurse to embrace and maintain cooperative relationships with all whom they meet. This includes other nurses or health practitioners as well as supporting staff members in clinical settings. If you decide to maintain a private practice, be sure to cooperate with government and other entities that govern your practice.

Holistic Nursing in Other Countries

If you are thinking of moving to another country, rest assured that you will be able to practice holistic medicine wherever you decide to go. Australia is one country that has embraced complementary medicine, and it experiences a more rapid growth each year. The reason for this growth comes mostly from the demand by the Australian public, 50 percent of who use herbal and complementary medicine. As in the United States, Australians have the strong desire to take a more active role in their wellbeing and health. Colleges all over Australia teach comprehensive courses in holistic medicine. The National Herbalist Association of Australia (NHAA) is the national entity for practicing herbalist. The NHAA sets minimum standards and provides accreditation to those who meet these requirements.

In the year 2005, over 45 percent of Denmark's 16 and over population received alternative medical treatment. The Danish Society for Medical Acupuncture consists of roughly 700 physicians. The chiropractic Association in Denmark has 300 members. This trend repeats itself worldwide in countries such as Germany, where three-quarters of their conventional treatment doctors also use complementary medicine; moreover, acupuncture treatments are used in 77 percent of the pain clinics in the country. Literally all over the world, holistic nurses like you are providing quality care with a holistic approach.

Income Potential

Since holistic nurses are trained in traditional medical techniques, they can expect to earn salaries comparable with other nurses. As with any profession, the setting, location, area and specific duties will dictate potential earnings. Typical salary for holistic nurses in the U.S. is $45,000 up to $95,000 per year. Salary increases with experience, but in many cases, an experienced holistic nurse earns a higher salary than the traditional nurse in the same setting. If your goal is to open your own holistic nursing practice, you can expect comparable earnings as your business develops and becomes established.

By all accounts, experienced holistic nurses are enjoying financial and professional success with their own nursing agencies and practices. Your experience in this industry provides you with an opportunity to take advantage of the current and future demand for your special skills.

Recent Holistic Medicine News

As a holistic nurse, you are embarking on a career that's on the cutting edge of modern healing. While definitely not a new medicine, holistic medicine is continuing to make strides that keep it the subject of recent news reports.

- **Harborside Health Center**

  Harborside Health Center, located in Oakland, California has been offering free holistic medical services, including medicines and education, for over five years. The founder, Steve DeAngelo, is a well known cannabis supporter who grew the Health Center into the largest medical cannabis dispensary in the United States with well over 90,000 registered patients. Recently, the center became the focus of a reality show, "Weed Wars." It is broadcast on the Discovery Channel. The founder has been quoted as saying that although he's not surprised that patients are in need of services provided by his center, he never imagined that he and his staff would star in a major cable television series.

- **United States Military Accepts Benefits of Holistic Medicine**

  The United States Department of Defense has recently recognized the benefits of alternative medicine. The Department has set aside billions of dollars to aid in researching in a variety of holistic based healing techniques. The Pentagon recently dedicated more than a five million dollar grant for research holistic techniques including meditation and acupuncture. The grant is set aside to develop these techniques to treat veterans who suffer Post Traumatic Stress Disorder. In addition, the U.S. Army awarded 4 million dollars for unconventional treatments for conditions such as anxiety, depression, substance abuse and PTSD. In all of these instances, early results show that these healing methods are showing promise in the treatment of military personnel and veterans.

- **Pacific College of Oriental Medicine Offers New Degree Program**

  Pacific College of Oriental Medicine (PCOM), a leading learning institution in the field of Traditional Chinese Medicine, has recently launched a brand new Bachelor degree program in holistic medicine. RN's who have already learned techniques such as Asian bodywork, herbal medicine, acupuncture and other TCM techniques can now advance their nursing careers by obtaining the new degree. Courses covered in the program include holistic theory and health and holistic healing modalities in addition to core leadership, science and research work.

Inspirational Stories

Join the thousands of holistic nurses who provide compassionate and skilled care to people suffering with illnesses. As you plan for your successful career, true life examples of excellent nursing in action can inspire you to keep going.

One successful holistic nurse came full circle in fulfillment of her childhood dreams. As a child, she engaged in pretend games in which she and her friends were nurses married to doctors. In her early teen years, she was inspired by reading about other real life nurses and volunteers. As she became older, she put aside her dream, feeling inadequate and lacking the confidence needed to study nursing. With the encouragement of her mother, also a nurse, she forged ahead and finished nursing school with honors. She is currently an elementary school nurse. She is fulfilled and proudly treats each child with a holistic approach, just as she dreamed as a child herself.

A compassionate nurse who considers himself a large "bearish" guy, had been known as the protector among his friends and family since childhood. As an adult, he performed jobs such as bouncer, body guard, and law enforcement officer. For 13 years, he worked as a gang investigator and eventually the negative environment took a toll on him. After testifying in a trial involving a horrible racial hate crime, his compassionate nature began to convince him to take a different career path. After working in a hospital emergency room for only 24 hours, he realized that nursing was his calling. He has been using his "unique and peculiar" nursing gifts for eight years to care for suffering human beings.

Do these nurses remind you of how passionate you are to serve as a holistic nurse? Let their stories encourage and inspire you in your own journey. The Nursing Inspiration Project website offers a wealth of information, encouragement and professional experience from nurses all around the world.

Chapter Review and Key Points to Remember

So, you've made the important decision to dedicate your career to serving yourself and others with the practice of holistic nursing. You should be congratulated for taking the first steps by following through with commitment to get the information you need.

In this chapter, you learned about the bravery of famous nurse Florence Nightingale. Her theories paved the way for patient care that treats the whole person, which we call holistic medicine today. Holistic nursing requires the knowledge, acceptance and practice of this treatment for the patient and nurse. It does not replace conventional medicine, but rather it complements medical treatment according to the desires of the patient.

Key Point - As a holistic nurse, it is important that you live a holistic lifestyle, not only for your own health and well being, but also to be able to effectively treat those in your care.

There are many facets of holistic nurses provided in this chapter. You learned that the nurse should be aware of the patient's beliefs and experiences in order to help to heal without forcing any type of treatment. These methods include physical and massage therapies and nutritional assessment and planning. However, non-traditional methods are widely used in this practice.

Key Point - You will be required to master unconventional treatment methods, including spiritual support. It is not your duty as a nurse to convince the patient of any belief or to accept any form of treatment.

Early in the chapter you read how holistic medicine was used to treat various illnesses and conditions. Chronic and acute symptoms, illness prevention as well as mental and emotional health are some of the fundamental uses for holistic medicine.

Key Point - Remember at all times that you are treating the whole person. Your goal should be to choose treatments that will help promote mental, physical and spiritual wholeness and healing.

Some characteristics of a good nurse include a caring personality, excellent communication skills and attention to detail. It is important that you remember to remain flexible, as people and situations constantly change on any given day.

Key Point - Your genuine passion for nursing is the major reason you are taking this important step. Remain honest in assessing your gifts and talents and never stop learning ways to improve your nursing skills.

Included in this chapter was information regarding nursing ethics. Issues regarding discrimination based on culture, race, sex and other life choices were covered. As a holistic nurse, your case should not be restricted by any of these issues.

Key Point - You, as a holistic nurse, are responsible for being a model in health care. All who come under your care should be treated with dignity and respect.

In addition to a passion for your work and natural ability, you learned that there are certain education requirements that must be met in order to practice. Holistic nurses have a bachelor's degree, and by far the majority of these are in nursing, but a few have the degree in other fields. However, all holistic nurses must have the appropriate holistic nursing certification in order to practice.

Key Point- If you are considering receiving your holistic nursing certification, research as many avenues as possible. Choose an accredited school or national certifications program, such as is offered by the American Holistic Nurses' Certification Corporation.

Holistic nurses can find employment in a variety of industries including hospitals, clinics and physicians offices. Many nurses set up their own practices and are able to make comparable salaries as nurses employed by others while owning their own business.

Key Point - Don't hesitate to begin your own nursing practice in order to enjoy the flexibility and freedom it brings. There is no doubt you can achieve this with careful planning, research and support.

There are several laws that govern the practice of holistic nursing. In addition to taking care of matters in setting up your practice such as location and marketing, it is important to familiarize yourself with these laws rather than risk your practice.

Key Point - Don't guess rules that relate to the scope of your practice. Every holistic nurse should study the Nurse Practice Act in order to be clear about the boundaries of their duties.

Summary

You are reading this material because you have made the decision to make holistic nursing not only a career, but also a life choice. Do not let anything deter you from reaching your goals of completing your education and starting your own practice. Remember to remain focused as well as open to any new possibilities you will encounter.

As you have learned, holistic nursing requires you, the nurse, to live a lifestyle conducive to wellness and wholeness. As such, make it a high priority to take care of your mind, body and spirit with a holistic approach. Take the necessary steps to maintain good physical health, employing holistic treatment as needed. Be sure to incorporate spiritual healing as needed to keep emotions in balance. A wealth of information is available to help guide your choices, including what educational and legal requirements you need in order to fulfill your life's purpose.

Don't try to go it alone; instead, accept helpful advice and support to help you reach your goals. Maintain confidence that you are a skilled professional fully up to the challenges of holistic nursing. Take the advice of the mother of holistic nursing, Florence Nightingale. Never "sacrifice the development" of your gifts for the sake of conventionality.

NURSING INFORMATICS

Using Nursing informatics to Both Profit and Heal

Nursing Informatics as a Profession

As a professional nurse, you have chosen a career that is diverse, lucrative and personally rewarding. Fortunately, you are virtually unlimited in the paths you can take to fulfill your career dreams. For many nurses like you, this means starting their own business within the nursing profession. Again, the choices for these ventures are limited only by the imagination.

Nursing informatics has continually evolved into a sub-discipline of the health care industry that is an excellent choice for nurses with the right skills, drive and entrepreneurial spirit that it takes to succeed. If you are a nurse who thrives in a role that integrates patient care with technology, perhaps you want to consider starting your own nursing informatics practice.

Nursing Informatics Overview and Definitions

Basically, nursing informatics focuses on the actual science of nursing combined with modern technology. It enhances the quality of the entire nursing practice by incorporating information science along with computer technology to achieve comprehensive health care goals. What this means for you, the professional nurse, is that by applying nursing informatics to your practices, you will be more efficient in communication, documentation and care of your clients.

The concept of nursing informatics began in the late 1960's. During this time, computer systems were introduced into the hospital setting and so called "computer nurses" were trained to operate them.

Nursing informatics as it stands today reflects the efforts of clinicians who were willing to expand their expertise in technology with their nursing education and skill in those early years.

The need for this health care specialty is based upon the increased involvement of nurses in the role they play in patient care. The health care industry, like all others, largely depends upon technology in order to function efficiently. As such, the nurse needs to be skilled at applying modern technology to diagnose, monitor and treat patients, in addition to the traditional medical attention and care needed. It is the efficient incorporation of information technology with nursing principles that is the foundation of nursing informatics.

Performing nursing informatics duties encompasses a wide variety of skills. There are several job titles that represent the scope of the nursing informatics specialty. These include:

- Clinical Applications Coordinator
- Clinical Analyst
- Nursing Informatics Specialist
- Nurse Systems Specialist
- Director of Clinical Informatics
- Clinical Informatics Manager

Although this dynamic nursing specialty dates back for more than three decades, you will find that there is no one final definition that describes nursing informatics in its entirety. This, in itself, gives you the freedom to create your own specialty nursing informatics practice that will provide excellent patient care. As you gather information about starting your own practice, it is a good idea to get a complete understanding of the scope and definition of this specialty to the extent it is available.

Nursing informatics is considered a distinct nursing specialty. The American Nursing Association (ANA) realized, however, that nurses specializing in informatics needed to define their practice. Therefore, the ANA "definition" for nursing informatics is more a guide that shapes the specialty. In addition, the definition is the national foundational element that is required by funding agencies to delineate projects and award money for research.

The basic definition by the ANA is that nursing informatics is a specialty that manages and communicates data, knowledge and information in a nursing practice by combining computer science with nursing and information science. Nursing informatics is the facilitator of this knowledge and information that provides support for patients and medical personnel to make decisions about the patient's health.

The tools that provide this support include informational structure that organizes data that is processed by computers and other technology. While this definition may seem lengthy and complicated, it is the goal of the ANA to provide a comprehensive explanation of the scope of the nursing informatics practice. As you prepare to begin your own business, you will come to appreciate the reasons for this, including the reasons outlined in the previous paragraph.

By most accounts, nursing informatics definitions have been categorized into three analytic themes over the past three decades:

- Information technology oriented. This, the earliest of nursing informatics definitions, focuses on the technology aspect of the practice. In its basic form, the definition outlined the relation of information technologies to the functions carried out by nurses that performed their duties. This detailed and broad definition even includes the education that nurses received in order to practice the nursing informatics discipline.

- Conceptually oriented. As this nursing specialty grew, the need to expand its scope also became apparent. As such, this further definition evolved in the late 1990's. The emphasis in this category is the actual purpose of such technology as it relates to the nursing practice. You will find that mastering the conceptual aspects of nursing informatics is just as, if not more, important than the technology itself. Many experts in this field agree that the conceptual and informational issues are primary when it comes to nursing informatics. Without such, they opine, the concepts of knowledge and nursing data cannot be combined into actual practice and movement in the science of nursing informatics.

- Role oriented. As the prevalence of nursing informatics grew, the need to clearly outline their roles became important. Eventually, the American Nursing Association made changes to the definition in order to assist in the creation of a certification examination in this specialty. The role oriented definition included the expansion of the nurse roles using tools, applications and processes that were continually developed.

Simply stated, the core components of nursing informatics are the nursing, computer and information sciences. As a nursing informatics professional, you will come to realize, however, that no definition encompasses the totality of this specialty. The organizing of these definitions into categories and core components merely serves to provide a structure to analyze the various aspects involved in nursing informatics. Revisions, as well as critiques of these definitions, continue to occur over the years as the specialty evolves.

Nursing Informatics Applications

Thus far, you have learned the basic theory behind the practice of nursing informatics. But what are the practical applications for this nursing specialty? As with any nursing specialty, the informatics nurse plays a vital role in the diagnosis, treatment and care of patients in their charge. As discussed, it is the integration of these duties with technology that distinguish this specialty. While not all inclusive, aspects of nursing informatics include the following:

• Collection of patient data

• Making availability of data easier

• Improve nursing capabilities to monitor quality measures

• Assisting in admission and discharge procedures

As an RN, you are well aware that the primary goal of a nurse is to provide the highest quality patient care and best nurse interaction as possible. Nursing informatics seeks to achieve these same goals with the use of computer technology.

Education, Training and Certification

Congratulations on your interest in expanding your nursing skills to include the information technology field! As a nurse, you have a proven record of being able to deliver quality health care utilizing hands on care combined with the use of the latest computer technology. This is extremely helpful since nursing informatics is by no means an entry level career. You have an understanding that computers and their applications are an essential part of health care and that the demand for nursing informatics continues to increase. As such, your plans to develop your own practice have begun at the optimal time.

Many universities offer informatics education through Bachelor degree nursing programs in the United States alone. Once nurses obtain their degree and other training, they are required to sit for the nursing informatics certification test. For current RN's who wish to begin a career in this specialty, continuing education programs can help them to prepare for the nursing informatics certification examination.

Nurses can also choose to pursue a Master of Science in Health Informatics at any number of universities in the country. For instance, the University of Illinois at Chicago offers students the opportunity to pursue such a degree online in a program that requires as little as 45 credit hours.

Nursing informatics specialist certification is given by the American Nurses Credentialing Center (ANCC) (http://www.nursecredentialing.org). Included among the topics that are covered in the examination are:

- Computer Technology

- Information and Database Management

- Theories

- Human Factors

- Professional Practice

- Trends and Issues

- System Support and Implementation

- System Design and Analysis

- System Evaluation and Testing

You can apply for the computer based test at any time during the year and from any location. Details regarding the examination can be found on their website. However, only active and licensed RN's with training in nursing informatics along with two years of nursing practice, including specific experience, can apply to take the exam. You will be able to find many resources with study guides, practice examinations and other reference material on the Internet to help you prepare to take your test.

It is also important that you check with your own state for nursing informatics certification in case there are additional requirements to those needed by ANCC.

Employment Industries

Nursing informatics specialists can find jobs in a number of different health care settings. Many of these professionals find work in the IT department in hospitals or doctor's offices. Others work in nursing homes and public or other types of health clinics. In addition to these traditional medical environments, nursing informatics specialists also work in the following industries:

- On staff consultation employees for insurance and other companies

- Training or administrative support workers for health related businesses such as pharmacies

- Working with vendors in sales, supply and systems support as a paid employee of a company

- On staff computer programmers who write and operate nursing computer applications

These nurses find rewarding and lucrative careers using their skills and talents to provide specialty health care. This chapter, however, is dedicated to helping you to start on the path of your very own nursing informatics practice and providing you with information to ensure its success.

The Nursing Informatics Specialist Entrepreneur

As a registered nurse, your options for business opportunities are endless. Thousands of RN's just like you have used their work experience, education and unique skills to develop successful, long term business ventures in healing and wholeness, educational, geriatric, legal, and forensic as well as hundreds of other related medical specialties.

Since you have decided to exercise your entrepreneurial dream and start your own nursing informatics practice, you will find that there are many specific areas within this practice that you can pursue. Many of these areas are similar to jobs that other nurses hold with other businesses. However, the difference is that you will be establishing your own business while exercising the same skills for which they are being paid.

Opportunities for RN's to open their own nursing informatics practice include:

• Consultation business for hospitals, insurance companies and other businesses.

• Administrative training company to offer education and training service for employees within a given business.

• Contracting computer programming or other skills.

• A systems support business for other companies to help them transition from traditional systems to computer based technology.

• A business that serves to facilitate the communication between technical and clinical staff.

Several steps will put help to you on the path to your business.

Identify your expertise. The initial stage of starting your practice includes recognizing and defining your unique expertise within the field. To help you to define your particular niche, you want to assess areas that apply to your nursing career up to this point. For instance, do you have years of patient safety or HIPAA regulation nursing experience? Or perhaps you have focused extensively on medical research during your career. It is important to identify whatever areas in which you have had a tendency to possess stronger skills, interest and experience. This information is essential in establishing you as an expert in a given area when you begin your nursing informatics practice.

Develop your business plan and make an honest financial assessment. As with any venture, a well laid out plan increases the chances of success. Develop a business plan that is solid and complete. Outline the services you plan to offer and provide a direction for the purpose of your business. Include details such as the fess you will charge and how your business will be represented.

Be sure to include a totally honest assessment of your financial picture both now, during the start up process and projected finances. This should include projected start up costs, such as building, utilities and tax implications. It should also include your plan for remaining financially viable as the business takes off. Most experts recommend that you keep liquid assets equal to six months in order to survive the initial period when your business will most likely not turn a profit.

Targeting and finding clients. As part of your business plan strategy, you need to begin to learn as much about your potential clients as possible. But first, you need to uncover where you will potentially find them. Many of the nursing informatics businesses we discussed will involve servicing the medical fields. Therefore, a large majority of your clients can be found in hospitals or other medical facilities such as nursing homes who need one or more of the areas of technical support that your business will office. Physicians' offices are other locations where you can find doctors who need someone to develop, run or train employees regarding the computer system or the medical technology used by the practice.

Insurance companies, government entities such as

Departments of Health and institutions of higher learning are also alternative locations for finding your future clients. Since you will have decided upon your niche by the time you reach this step, you will be more aware of which of these locations will offer you the most potential for finding just the right clients.

There are also online resources that provide the opportunity to purchase contact information about potential clients. Info USA (http://www.infousa.com) is one such company that offers quality business sales leads for more than 14 million businesses looking for customers.

Marketing your business. Once you have determined who you wish to target, you must pull out all stops to market yourself and your business services. Take advantage of all available resources that will shed the best light possible on your company and its services to as many people as possible. PR Health Care Communications (www.PRHealthCareCommunications.com) is a company that offers expert public relations services for nurses and other medical professionals. The company will market your company and create a business presence for your company that will establish a sense of professionalism, trust, credibility and competency to all potential clients. They will help you to brand your business using marketing tools such as business cards, letterhead and other printed materials. In addition, they will help you to generate interest through printed media, radio and television advertising.

In today's world, no business is complete without securing an Internet presence. You will want a professionally designed website that reflects your services. While most every new business launches a website, some newer entrepreneurs are not aware that, in order for the website to stand out among millions, it must be search engine optimized. Search engine optimization is a complex process that involves ensuring that a website comes up at the top of the list in a search. If not properly optimized, a website will become lost in the World Wide Web. Ideally, you do not want to skimp on this important aspect of promoting your business. Hire professional web marketing companies, especially those that are geared to promote websites in the health care industry. Medical Marketing SEO (www.MedicalMarketingSEO.com) has a proven track record of delivering top search engine optimization for businesses in the health care industry.

Participate in self promotion. In order to establish yourself as an expert in your field, make sure that you build both history and a business presence by being proactive in your own advertising. Even before you officially open your business, tell people about your impending practice and what you intend to offer clients. Always be prepared to deliver an accurate and articulate presentation in a professional manner. Your reputation will be your lifeline, so don't over inflate the scope of your services. At the same time, do not hesitate to take an opportunity to tell people about your business and encourage them to tell others. A large number of your clients will be word of mouth referrals that result from encounters such as this. Present yourself as the caring expert in the field that you are and let your enthusiasm show through in your delivery of information. Always keep your business cards, flyers and other information readily available to pass out to anyone who expresses an interest in your business.

Practice approaching people about your business and answering questions that may arise on a regular basis. Your goal is to be able to present yourself as an expert in a manner that demonstrates your knowledge but is understandable to the listener. Having the ability to market your own practice will prove to be a crucial aspect of promoting your business.

Among other means to promote your own business, you should consider running classified ads. You can find hundreds of industry related free classified advertising websites on the Internet. These sites allow you to put a link to your website and other contact information in the appropriate industry category. Another way you can promote your business is to volunteer to write for trade magazines in exchange for a plug for your business. This option is also a way to impress readers with your knowledge about medicine, nursing, informatics or related topics. Other websites such as Squidoo and Living Social accept articles from business owners that provide the opportunity to showcase company information.

Earning Expectations

The opportunities are endless for nurses like you to develop private practices in the nursing informatics industries. Statistics show that registered nurses working for other companies are enjoying excellent income and other benefits. As a business owner, you can expect similar or even greater success as you build your business.

By all accounts, nursing informatics is a field of medicine that is expected to continue to grow into the future. Among the many reasons for this fact is that the health care and information technology industries are among the highest ranking occupational fields. The U.S. Bureau of Labor Statistics has predicted a 22 percent increase in employment over the next ten years for nursing informatics specialists. For registered nurses employed by various companies, salary expectation varies depending on a number of factors; which include:

- Work experience. Registered nurses with at least 20 years of experience can expect to earn the highest salaries as nursing informatics specialists. On average, nurses with one year working experience earn between $59,000 and $73,000 annually, depending on location and other factors. By comparison, nursing informatics specialists with more years of experience earn increasing salaries for every year they have worked, up to $80,000 or more each year depending on the number of years of experience.

- Geographical location. As with any industry, salaries can vary depending on the region where the company is located; in addition to the number of years in work experience. In the United States, nursing informatics specialists in the state of Georgia earn about $60,000 to $80,000 salary yearly. Pennsylvania nursing informatics specialists earn, on average, a starting wage of $68,000. The state of Massachusetts pays nursing informatics specialists the highest average salaries in the nation, with salaries of close to $69,000 to over $102,000 annually.

- Some reports indicate that male nurses make a higher salary than female nursing informatics specialists, as much as $30,000 higher each year.

- Company size. In the United States, the size of the company does not appear to affect the earnings potential of nursing informatics specialists by a large margin. Current statistics place companies with 20,000 employees as paying salaries that fall within the middle range of $66,000 to $76,000 each year.

The above information can serve as a guide to what you can expect to earn or the fees you can charge your own clients. Other factors that can affect salary include the continuing education and training that the professional chooses to pursue after employment. As a business owner, you have more control of your earning potential. You are in the fortunate position of having flexibility with regard to wages, benefits, location and the amount of hours you work. In addition, you can decide how small or large you desire to grow your business. This freedom is why so many others like you start their own practices each year.

The Future of Nursing Informatics

Again, you have chosen to pursue a career that will affect the health care industry long into the future. In fact, informatics technology and medicine will continue to merge and integrate as the demand dictates. Industry analysts outline several areas that will require the need for well trained nursing informatics specialists. Some of these areas are in the infancy stages and are expected to evolve and grow. Others are still in the planning stages and will become state of the art informatics technology in upcoming years.

Increased use of bio-metric cards. Electronic medical identity cards contain information about a person's medical conditions and medical history. They are the new level of medical identity bracelets or printed cards that people who have conditions such as diabetes or heart disease have kept in their possession for many years. These electronic cards are scanned by EMS personnel and medical personnel in the hospital emergency room. The future of these cards includes imbedding more detail regarding the patient into the card. This includes instant verification of the patient's identity by scanning the eye, fingerprint and even the DNA makeup. This data is sent to various departments in the hospital that will be used in patient care, including the pharmacy, dieticians and the patient's bedside.

The evolution of the bio-metric card includes the ability to upload the information to the hospital so that it is accessed by hospital personnel via computer before the patient arrives. Medical personnel will know about allergies, medical conditions and medication, blood type and even insurance information instantly from the EMS team uploading such data from the card to the hospital. Already on the market are new subscription based medical cards that allow people to access their own medical records via USB cards.

As a nursing informatics specialist, you are in a position to use your expertise in the training, design, and management of biomedical cards in the hospital setting as they continue to evolve.

The utilization of tele-nursing and telemedicine in the home setting. Today, hospital patients are being discharged earlier and with more frequency due to advances in medicine. Many of these patients are still in the process of healing and may require home care as they do so. Nursing informatics can be a key tool in monitoring health care for patients including prescription and other home care assistance. Your nursing informatics practice can be a resource for those recovering patients to design, maintain and monitor the technology that is the bridge to the hospital and medical personnel assigned to their care.

Education. There are current proposals to include nursing informatics as a requirement in the nursing school curriculum. The introduction of this specialty to the beginning nurse is said to, at the very least, provide them with an overall view of what is fast becoming a necessary part of nursing. While some disagree with nursing informatics as a prerequisite of a nursing degree, many others believe that it should be a requirement in these times of ever changing computer technology in the health care industry.

Implementation and expansion of clinical technology. This is truly an exciting time catch the wave of medically related technology. Now and into the future, the practice of nursing informatics will play a key role in helping businesses and other organization make decisions regarding the purchase and implementation of technology. The practice will continue to affect other departments such as information technology and administration. It will also be a means to improve the quality of medical care including saving time and money for the patient.

The entire health care team for a patient will become increasingly joined in a concerted effort to provide top quality, efficient and cost saving care as the industry expands. The more you stay on top of the latest developments, the more you increase your chances of becoming an expert in this field.

Summary

It is a well known fact that the medical industry, and practically every other industry, has become increasingly dependent upon technology in this digital age. In the nursing sector, you have most likely seen such technology grow in patient care from remote devices, smart beds automatic data capture, and other functions in the medical setting. You are already ahead of the curve by making plans to develop and market a nursing informatics practice. You can start right away by implementing the suggestions outlined in this chapter as well as utilizing available tools that will become a part of your success.

To put your education and skills to the best use possible, continue to acquire your information technology skills throughout the process. Focus on database management, computer language, and system design in order to be prepared to offer your clients a wide variety of services.

Learn as much as possible about the nursing informatics specialty by reading textbooks, journals, and keeping up with the latest news about this specialty. Expand your knowledge by reading information about the nursing field in general, such as the book "The Nurse Expert". This book contains comprehensive information about how to use your nursing expertise in any area to build rewarding and profitable businesses. Attend as many conferences as you can for further knowledge and to network with other nurses and medical professionals in this field.

Along the same lines, invest in yourself and your future business by joining professional organizations dedicated to nursing informatics. This will help you to know which areas to focus on in preparation for your certification. Many RN's choose to purse graduate school to increase their visibility as a nursing informatics professional. This option will also give you more credibility as an expert when you open your practice.

Ensure that you are fully prepared to do your best on your nursing informatics certification examination by doing careful research and study before you take the test.

Plan your business strategy well. Make an honest assessment regarding your financial situation and prepare for the inevitable income shortage that will occur with any fledgling business. Perform due diligence by thoroughly researching the earning potential you can expect throughout your years in practice.

Don't neglect getting the word out regarding yourself and your business venture. Volunteer to do seminars, write articles or any other means to advertise. Take advantage of companies that will help to promote your business in a professional manner such as PR Healthcare Communications and Medical Marketing SEO. These businesses are fundamental in helping RN's like you to put your best foot forward when starting a nurse related practice. They have helped countless nursing professionals with public relations, advertising and website design and optimization.

Keep informed about the latest advances in nursing informatics technology. This will not only keep your services relevant, but will increase your position as an expert in your field.

Did you know that nurses outrank medical doctors by 15 percent as medical professionals? In a Gallup survey conducted in December of 2010, a whopping 85 percent of the people who responded viewed nurses as having a high or very high standard of ethics. This ranking put nurses among the top rated professions along with clergy, grade school teachers, police officers and other professionals. As such, you are among an elite group of people who how the power to influence the practice of medicine.

As a trusted medical professional, you are in a position to use your practice to meet the challenge, both now and into the future, of advancing the role of the nurse in changing and advancing the health industry as a whole.

SMOKING CESSATION

The Role of the Nurse in Smoking Cessation Coaching

As a medical professional, you are on the front line in the fight for people to achieve and maintain the best health possible. You have seen firsthand the effects that disease, eating habits and lifestyle can have on patients, in both negative and positive ways.

As you know, smoking is one of the leading causes of illness, disease and death. In this chapter, we will cover how you, as a nurse, can help people to stop smoking and also play a part in the reducing the number of new smokers through preventative measures. Additionally, you will learn how you can live your dream and start, maintain and profit from utilizing your medical expertise and experience, compassion and various resources to start a smoking cessation coaching practice of your very own.

Smoking Statistics

The sad statistics all across the globe are a testament to the need for smoking cessation coaching. The negative effects of smoking do not discriminate based upon age, race, gender or geographical location. Below are just a very few of the startling figures that underscore the need for smoking intervention and prevention. They include:

- There are over 5 million deaths worldwide that are attributed to tobacco use. According to the Center for Disease Control, the next couple of decades will see an increase to over 8 million deaths each year if the current trends continue.

- In the UK alone, over 120,000 citizens died from smoking related causes in the year 2004, making it one of the biggest public health threats in the area.

- By some estimates, $50 billion dollars is spent on health costs due to smoking in the United States. It is considered to have a more lethal impact on public health than a combination of automobile accidents, AIDS, homicides and suicides, fires and drug overdoses combined.

- Despite devastating statistics, the tobacco industry spent over $12 billion on the promotion and advertising of their products, an average of over $30 million each day.

- In addition to deaths related to smoking, habitual tobacco use is responsible for heart disease, lung cancer, emphysema, pneumonia and chronic bronchitis. Smokers are at an extreme risk of stroke, hypertension and aneurysms. A person who smokes is three times more likely to develop Type 2 (non insulin dependent) diabetes. Pregnant women who smoke risk delivering babies with low birth weight, which can lead to a number of health problems for the infant. Smoking can reduce life expectancy by some 20 years in many cases and about 14 years on average.

- Second hand smoke also poses grave danger to non smokers because it contains equally dangerous contaminates, which can be even more dangerous since the smaller particles go deeper into the lungs. Passive smoke causes about 46,000 deaths every year from heart disease among nonsmoking adults in the United States. Infants exposed to second hand smoke suffer from asthma attacks and other respiratory problems, ear infections and a higher risk of sudden infant death syndrome.

Additional risks include fertility issues such as difficulty in getting pregnant in women and a reduction of sexual function in men. Deaths from Sudden Infant Death Syndrome are at a higher risk in smoking mothers. Some cosmetic effects of smoking include breath and body odor, stained teeth and an increase in facial wrinkling.

You have chosen well for this business opportunity since there is never a shortage of clients that need help to quit smoking. There are over one billion people around the world that smoke; the United States has close to 50 million alone. Your coaching will assist smokers to identify why they smoke and lead them to change their thinking and actions to quit.

As a smoking cessation coach, you are in a position to help people take one of the most important steps in improving their health. Your business can provide effective tools and health care assistance needed for smokers to make major changes in their lives. Your smoking cessation business will also be a source of inspiration and encouragement that will guide smokers toward enjoying the many advantages of living smoke free.

The Benefits of Quitting

You are most likely aware of the many benefits your future clients can enjoy from stopping their smoking habit. Sharing these benefits will be most helpful to you in convincing them that they are making an extremely wise choice that will improve not only their physical health, but their emotional and mental health as well.

Your advice will include providing your clients with factual information about the prospect of reversing many physical conditions within the body that starts as early as 20 minutes after they stop smoking. It is after this time when the pulse rate and blood pressure begin to return to normal. Many smokers are not aware that after 72 hours of not smoking, the whole body tests 100 percent free of nicotine and 90 percent nicotine chemical free. Information such as this that you share with your clients will provide the incentive for them to continue in their efforts remain smoke free longer and longer until they have quit entirely.

Other positive benefits that increase with time include reduction in cravings within ten days and a giant leap in the chance of complete recovery within two weeks. Oral blood circulation also returns to levels similar to non smokers within this time frame. Starting at two weeks and up until three months, lung function, circulation, chronic cough and heart attack risk has dropped. After one year, the risk of heart attack has dropped by less than half and the long list of health benefits continue to rise in subsequent years of smoke free living.

Sharing the emotional and financial benefits that can be achieved from quitting will also be useful to the people whom you care for in your practice. For instance, this habit oftentimes causes severe emotional distress caused by the smoking urges themselves. These urges cause distraction, interruption in daily activities and other issues to the extent that people become tense and frustrated, rather than relaxed, which can have an adverse affect on their family and working life. The seemingly never ending cycle of strong urges followed by temporary relief can make life miserable for some smokers, similar to other addictions. Guilt associated with smoking (about loved ones concern for health, smoking around children or elderly, rising cost of cigarettes, etc.) is also a real concern that some people may not even be aware of.

Studies indicate that a great many smokers have feelings of depression, anger and even confusion related their addiction. Many smokers are alleviated of such distractions, concern regarding financial issues and negative emotions when they stop smoking. As a nurse, you are an ideal candidate to help clients navigate through this maze of emotions.

Anti-Smoking Initiatives

For decades, nurses have played an enormous role in the treatment and reduction of diseases relating to smoking. They also contribute to reversing the rising numbers of smokers around the world through education and coaching of smokers and those who are at risk of starting to smoke, such as adolescents. Nurses also are among the most active groups that participate in campaigns and initiatives designed to address the many issues that relate to tobacco use, which include:

- The Campaign for Tobacco-Free Kids

  This non-profit organization was founded in 1996 and has become prominent as a worldwide fighter to reduce tobacco use around the globe. The organization's work includes advocating for changes in public policies to prevent young people from smoking. Among their other work are initiatives to educate and prevent secondhand smoke and programs to help smokers stop tobacco use.

- Lung Cancer Awareness Month

  This campaign began in 1995 as Lung Cancer Awareness Day and has since spread to include numerous activities. Officially, Lung Cancer Awareness Month is in November, yet participation and activities are continued year round. These include bringing attention to the disease through special events, books, articles and other writings, Internet promotion and the issuance of Proclamations. Vigils which include hundreds of events over three continents, biking, walking and other marathons and memorials to victims of the disease are just a few of the activities that occur during Lung Cancer Awareness Month.

- Media and Advertising

  The anti-smoking movement has made leaps and bounds in its efforts to provide advertisements that discourage smoking. Huge marketing campaigns in recent years have openly revealed the negative effects that smoking has on smokers and those that inhale second hand smoke. Television commercials, radio announcements and visual marketing tools such as posters and videos get more creative every year to urge people to quit smoking and promote the benefits of doing so.

- Government participation

  Governments in the United States and other countries are becoming more active in educating citizens about the negative effects of tobacco use. Among these recent efforts in the United States is the Food and Drug Administration's pledge of $600 million for tobacco education. The money will be spread over a five year period with the goal of reducing disease and death resulting from tobacco. In 2003, The World Health Organization adopted the Framework Convention on Tobacco Control, a treaty signed by 168 countries. It was among the fastest ratified treaties in the history of the United Nations. It is designed to protect people now and into the future from the long list of consequences that result from tobacco use and exposure to its smoke.

The U.S. Department of Human Services, Office of the Surgeon General, is a governmental source with a wealth of information for smokers and those who are helping them to quit. The website is filled with related news including new initiatives as well as valuable clinician and consumer materials and other resources.

Nurses are a Perfect Fit as Smoking Cessation Coaches

Just by virtue of being a nurse, you are seen by others as a person of authority, possessing education and knowledge in addition to having a compassionate nature. You are a respected professional whose advice will, in most cases, be respected and have an impact on the success of a smoker. These facts have been substantiated by studies that included smokers of all ages from a variety of locations. Among the conclusions reached by these studies include:

- The rate of success of smokers who quit independently is less than 3 percent. The likelihood that a person will quit smoking is marginally increased when provided advice by a nursing professional, since nurses are generally regarded as authoritative role models with regard to health. The nurse provides coaching, counseling and support that medications alone cannot provide, such as addressing environmental influence, smoking triggers and other issues.

• According to the International Council of Nurses, they have a distinct advantage over others when it comes to providing smoking cessation services. The experience that nurses acquire in advising patients (including advising them to quit smoking) in the hospital setting has equipped them with specific skills that are essential in helping people to stop smoking.

• Nurses, as opposed to non medical personnel, are better able to communicate the health risks and benefits to people who desire to stop smoking. Throughout the career of a nurse, they have acquired education and first hand awareness about smoking and its effects on health, which they can share with people to encourage them to give up the habit. This includes providing people with information about various options and aids that other smokers have used.

How Nurses Assist Smokers to Stop Smoking

The first step to stop smoking, or to cease any other addictive behavior, is a willingness to do so. Part of your job will be to determine what, if any, is the patient's motivation for quitting if they desire to do so. There are basic steps that move people toward the path of living a tobacco free lifestyle. These begin with smokers who have no intention to stop smoking up to those who are thinking about doing so. At some point, a person willing to quit will begin preparing by setting a date to quit, smoking less and other actions. The ultimate goal is the cessation of the habit and consistent maintenance, including regular follow up to avoid relapse.

As a nursing coach, you will possess the ability to assist people throughout their journey who have a true desire to stop smoking. In the majority of cases, these will be people who have tried to quit on their own without success. They will be eager to get help from the services that your smoking cessation coaching services will offer. Among the tools you will provide to your clients include:

*   Assess each client on their smoking status, which includes their level of nicotine dependence. One standard measurement that is used to assess smokers is called the Fagerstrom Test of Nicotine Dependence (FTND). Smokers are asked questions such as how much, when and where they smoke and whether they smoke when they first wake up. They are also asked if they find it difficult to not smoke in places where tobacco use is prohibited such as movie theaters and other public places. The answers to the questions are rated and used to determine the level of dependence within the range of very low to very high dependence.

*   Supply the client with information about health risks to not only themselves, but to their loved ones. Although most smokers are aware of how their habit is affecting their own health, the prospect of improving the health of their family members may be added incentive to their quitting.

*   Provide various levels of mental and emotional support including advice and listening to some of the issues that are related to the tobacco addiction

of the client. It can also be helpful to your practice if you decide to share your own struggles with regard to past smoking or other unhealthy habits that you have overcome. This builds a sense of trust with your client and serves as inspiration in his or her own life.

- Monitor progress and suggest coping techniques while addressing problems.

- Develop individual strategies for each client that will lead to successful smoking cessation.

- Provide information regarding medications or other stop smoking aids.

As the owner of your own practice, you can create coaching techniques and make other decisions that will be unique to your business. You will have the freedom to choose when, how and where you will provide coaching. This, along with many other factors, will make your business stand out and become successful.

Opportunities that Exist for Nurses in this Field

This business involves creating a rewarding and profitable company created from your heart for seeing people become healthy and whole. There are many reasons nurses like you find success with their own smoking cessation businesses. Your education, skills and expertise will be combined with this natural ability to create a niche that will make a huge difference in people's lives.

There are countless options for you to use as a foundation to build and maintain a healthy business of your own if you keep your eye out for possibilities. For instance, pregnant women who smoke make excellent potential clients since most are concerned with not only their health, but the health of their baby. In addition to running a business with a client base that you coach in person, there are other alternatives that nurses use that result in successful business ventures. Below are a few brief descriptions of opportunities to start your own smoking cessation coaching practice.

Speaking engagements. You can share your knowledge as an expert on smoking cessation by becoming a speaker at a various events. Groups and organizations often hire life coaches to inspire and encourage attendees at their health related events. Many nurses promote themselves as open to traveling nationally or internationally on a full time basis as an expert speaker on smoking and other topics.

Consultation services. Doctor's or dentist's offices, clinics, non-profit organizations that promote public health and schools are just a few places that you can offer consultation services. These may need you to provide them with information about smoking cessation for classes they conduct. Alternatively, they may want to refer people to you who wish to quit smoking. In either event, the field is wide open for professional experts (especially in the health care industry) to promote healthier lifestyles including smoking cessation.

Remote coaching. Some nurses operate a telephone help line for people who are trying to quit smoking. This line is usually open to callers 24 hours a day to get advice, resources or any other help they may need. You can also coach over the Internet in one of several ways. Some nurses run a website that has information about smoking cessation as well as "live chat" during certain hours of the day. Others deliver periodic topical presentations to paid clients over the Internet and/or hold teleconferences for people who are trying to quit smoking.

Writing. It is possible to become an expert smoking cessation coach by writing books or articles on the subject. On the Internet, online magazines, healthy living websites and others are looking for professionals who can provide informative content on health related issues including how, why and when to quit smoking. Combining this with writing your own real life stories, books or newsletters can help you grow a profitable business.

Other business ideas include teaching as well as distribution and sale of products that help people to quit smoking, such as smokeless cigarettes and nicotine lozenges. There are no limits to the exciting possibilities that lay ahead for you in your career as a smoking cessation coach. Are you motivated to start your very own business program but unsure where to start?

You can receive all the training and information you need so that you are fully equipped to offer smoking cessation counseling with programs provided by RN Health Coaching services found at:

www.HealthCoachNursingJobs.com.

RN Health Coach

RN Health Coach.com is a leading source of comprehensive training and support for nurses like you who have a desire to establish, operate and market their own health coaching services. RN Health Coach (RNHealthCoach.com) incorporates years of experience and research in the health care industry to guide nurses through the process of providing personal health coaching services to individuals struggling with various medical and/or behavioral conditions. Weight loss, worksite wellness and smoking cessation are among the successful programs that we have had the privilege of helping nurses to develop.

You are reading this material because you are a nurse who has the skills to interact with patients and the ability to approach healthcare management in a proactive manner. Allow yourself to combine these skills with your desire to take control of your destiny by establishing a coaching practice of your own. You can be assured that your coaching program will be fully prepared to deliver all of the elements that will lead to its success. The site will equip you to educate and motivate your clients to achieve their goals through proven tools and techniques.

The approach to coaching. The focus in smoking cessation coaching is first identifying and then changing certain mindsets and behaviors that tie people up in the smoking cycle. The service will show you the methods used to go directly to the client's beliefs with regard to smoking. Addressing the attitude of the smoker about quitting will reveal any negative thoughts that could lead to defeat. As a coach, you will then help the smoker to eventually replace thoughts and behaviors with more constructive thinking and actions that result in quitting.

Methodology and Tools.

HealthCoachNursingJobs.com will train you how to help your clients stop smoking by using proven effective techniques to guide them through each step in their goal. For instance, in order to formulate a plan specific to each individual, there are specific areas you will need to explore to get an overall picture of the smoker.

Initially, you will need to assess the level of the smoker's dependency on nicotine and to what degree they are ready to stop smoking. Questionnaires such as the Fagerstrom Test of Nicotine Dependence are used for this purpose, and you will be introduced and trained in using this assessment tool. At that point, it will be your job as a health care professional and coach is to provide direct and clear advice to your client to stop smoking, along with clear reasons why it would be in their best interest to do so.

RN Health Coach will equip you with the skills to assess the smoker's motivation for quitting by teaching and training you how to use the five stages of behavior change. This includes training in motivational interviewing and supporting the client as they progress through these stages. They will train you how to address issues such as ambivalence, excuses for not quitting and avoiding triggers that lead people to smoke. Through RN Health Coach training, you will gain a working knowledge how to use your nursing background to provide advice about Nicotine Replacement Therapy and medications and how to determine whether they would be helpful for your client.

Follow up. Once the ultimate goal is reached, you will need to continue to be a source of support for your client. Your coaching will continue to provide tools and techniques for intervention, positive support when the client quits smoking and follow up as needed. This follow up is needed in order to determine how your client is progressing in areas of cravings, withdrawal symptoms and medication use. As a nurse coach during the follow up phase, you will be able to provide the listening ear that clients need to discuss any challenges they may be experiencing, as well as offer encouragement and suggest resources.

Don't hesitate to contact RN Health Coaching to get further information about our programs that assist nurses with realizing their dreams of becoming health coaching business owners. Once you have your business up and running, they will also provide you with a wide range of services to promote and market your business, which are discussed later in this chapter.

Success Stories

Tobacco use is an addiction, as well as a habit, that is extremely hard to break. Smokers that have help with quitting have a much higher success rate than those who try to go it alone. Countless ex-smokers are willing to share their testimonies about how they were able to stop with the help of cessation coaching in a variety of formats including in person, telephone and online. Below are just a few inspirational, successful stories that have been the result of cessation counseling.

A 69 year old woman from Vermont smoked since she was 15 years old. After trying for many years to quit without success, she was about to give up giving up when she was diagnosed with a form of breast cancer. This diagnosis gave her the incentive to try to quit again and she reached out for coaching to help her stop. The coaching provided the tools and encouragement she needed to give up her long term tobacco habit. She now reports that she is both cancer and smoke free because of the help she received from the coach team, to whom she gives full credit for her success.

Corporations that have hired health coaches to help employees quit smoking have reaped enormous returns on their investment. One corporation in Los Angeles estimates that they have had a 3 to 1 return on their investment over the course of three years, not only in terms of costs, but in savings from lower health care, disability and higher productivity. The owners of the company highly recommend other business owners to hire coaches to achieve their own smoke free workplaces.

Earnings Potential for Wellness Coaches

Each year, millions of desperate people seek advice and support regarding their physical and emotional health. Because of this, nurses and other professionals develop careers that entail helping people in areas such as stress management, healthy eating and lifestyle changes among many others. Smoking cessation coaches are among the many types of wellness coaches that are very popular and lucrative today.

The average earnings for a few of these businesses are outlined below. This information is presented as a guideline, as every business will earn more or less, depending on several issues including the type of practice, experience and geographical location. As the owner of your business, your earnings potential depends on the amount of time you desire to spend in your practice among a long list of other factors.

- Corporate Wellness Programs. Large corporations sometimes hire a person who serves as a wellness coach for the employees of the company. This coach motivates the employees to improve their overall health and wellbeing by planning health fairs, providing information about healthier lifestyles and offering health counseling. In the United States, corporate wellness managers typically earn approximately $60,000 to $80,000 annually.

- Disease education and management. These wellness coaches usually address specific diseases such as diabetes and other chronic conditions. Coaching includes prevention for people who may be at risk as well as current patients. Also included is comprehensive education about the disease or condition and how lifestyle, eating habits and other factors affect the condition. Certified disease management coaches and educators earn a median salary of $65,000 a year.

- Fitness coaching. Fitness coaching includes nutritional guidance, exercise and living an overall healthy lifestyle. Personal trainers can also fall into this category. Fitness coaches that have certification or a degree can expect to earn approximately $60,000 a year, depending on how many hours they work and the region in which they practice.

Overall, if your smoking cessation practice is in a larger city your earning potential is higher. Other factors that affect earnings are whether the coaching is face to face, over the phone, in group settings or one on one. It is a good idea to research the cost of similar programs in your area in order to gauge what you should charge for each session. Then take into account any other services you will be offering and adjust your fees accordingly.

The Business Plan

Your solid business plan will include outlining your services, targeting your clients and providing an accurate financial assessment. Take your time to define the nature and scope of the services you intend to provide; this will be the foundation of your entire business. Seek out places that you think will most likely need your services to investigate the potential for clients.

In assessing your finances, be sure to include an estimate of what your start up costs will be. These costs will vary greatly depending on several things such as the services you provide, whether you will coach clients in person at your own establishment, the costs for you to travel to your clients if you will go to their location, or associated costs if you will provide coaching remotely over the telephone or Internet. Be sure to factor in your current financial situation and make sure you have money to live on while your business is established.

You will invest the time and research needed to carefully map out each of these important areas in detail. Once complete, you will be ready to take the next step in your business - getting the word out about your smoking cessation coaching business.

Marketing and Promotion of Your Business

It is essential that your business is promoted accurately, consistently and in a professional manner. No matter how great your services are, an inadequate marketing campaign can mean that only you and your close friends are aware the business even exists. We have many years of experience assisting nursing professionals like you in getting the word out about their health coaching and other businesses. PR Health

Care Communications (www.PRHealthCareCommunications.com) provides public relations services in order to establish your company as a solid business presence. Your unique brand can be presented to the public with the aid of marketing tools and printed media, as well as radio and television interviews and advertising.

We also actively engage in lead generation for the program. Websites such as www.StopSmokingCessationPrograms.com direct smokers who are looking for help to quit smoking to resources such as RNHealthCoach.com , where they can find information about smoking cessation coaches in their area.

The fast paced technological world of today also demands that businesses secure a presence on the World Wide Web. An interactive, content rich website is essential for this purpose. However, in order for your website to be seen by millions it must be search engine optimized. Search engine optimization is the key to ensuring that your business comes up among the first when a visitor is searching the Internet for a smoking cessation coach.

Our company, Medical Marketing SEO (www.MedicalMarketingSEO.com), specializes in placing medical related websites in the top results of major search engines.

There is no such thing as too much promotion, and you will prove to be a primary marketing tool for your business. Take every opportunity you can to let others know that you are an expert smoking cessation coach with a thriving practice. Protect your reputation by being professional at all times and in every way, including your appearance, presentation and marketing materials such as business cards. Become even more proactive by placing your business information in relevant classified ads on the Internet; there are literally hundreds of these that you can place ads in for free. You can also promote your business by opening business accounts on social websites such as Facebook and/or writing about your business in blogs such as Squidoo.

Chapter Review and Key Points to Remember

The nursing profession puts you in a position where you have major influence in the health of patients. As a smoking cessation coach, you have a profound effect on the minds of smokers that can change their health and entire lives for the better. Since tobacco is a product that kills half of the consumers who buy it, your contribution will also save many lives.

Key point - Smoking affects nearly every person on the face of the planet.

Over five million people die as a result of tobacco use in some form. People who do not smoke, as well as those who inhale secondhand smoke, are also greatly affected by its use on various levels. In addition, smoking has an adverse financial affect on people who may not fall into either of these categories. The astronomical medical costs related to smoking result in overall increases in medical insurance and health care for smokers and non smokers alike.

Key point - People who smoke can see almost immediate positive results.

Twenty short seconds after a smoke, the body starts to heal itself by lowering blood pressure and pulse rate. Major health restoration takes place starting with 3 days through a lifetime of smoke free living. People who remain smoke free can look forward to improved circulation and lung function, absence of the classic "smokers cough" and a long list of other improvements, including reducing the risk of heart attack by half or more. As a smoking cessation coach, you can share this information with your clients, which may be the incentive they need to stay on track.

Key point - Your participating in anti smoking initiatives can make a difference.

You are in an excellent position to become a voice for health change. There are a wide variety of activities in which you can join others as a united front against smoking.

Key point - Your options as a smoking cessation coach are unlimited.

Many nurses before you have been successful as coaches because they have integrated their love of the profession with their innate talents and interests. For instance, if you have a gift for writing, you can focus your business on sharing your expertise through books, magazine articles and other writings, including speeches and anti smoking advertising copy.

Key point - You have worked very hard to reach this point in your career as a nurse.

Don't make the mistake, as some have, of moving too quickly through the initial steps of starting your business in your enthusiasm to get going. Take time to carefully research the market in the area you wish to practice. Take note of potential sources for clients and develop ways to pitch your business to these sources. Methodically prepare your business plan so that you can clearly see your vision and make adjustments if necessary.

Don't shy away from being brutally honest about finances. Look into legal and tax implications that relate to your business, costs for fees or documentation, operating costs, the cost for marketing and promotion, and your personal finances and any other money matter. A carefully laid out plan will pay off tremendously when your business takes off, which it is sure to do eventually.

Summary

In actuality, no further proof is needed to illustrate to the entire world that immediate and continual action to stop smoking is necessary. Health care professionals see the devastation caused each and every day. Research reveals alarming statistics that rise with each passing year. The promising news is that some countries, including the United States, are seeing a small decrease, or at least a leveling off, in the number of smokers each year.

Sadly, however, the world is still at risk of a resurgence of new smokers starting at even younger ages than in the past, which is why this will be a continuing hard fought battle. We congratulate the efforts of nurses such as you who have decided to pull up their sleeves and take an aggressive stance in helping people to free themselves from this addiction. Your decision will be rewarded with a lifetime of fulfillment, prosperity and sense of great accomplishment in knowing you have made a huge difference.

CONCLUSION

As you finish reading through this book, you should feel as though you have a clear grasp of what is going on both in the current nursing field and what you need to overcome any roadblocks and succeed. As the nursing field changes and more and more nurses are unhappy, there has begun to be a shift in the potential for registered nurses.

Remember for a second the reasons why nurses are unhappy with their current bedside jobs, including:

• Being overworked.

• Being underpaid.

• Being underappreciated.

• Stressful working hours.

• Lack of job security.

• Becoming burned out.

While this is the bad news about the current state of the nursing field, the good news is that you have a chance to change your life. You have not only found this book, but read and understood the information it contains. This information means that you are able to overcome these issues in the nursing field and find a way to use your degree and experience in a way that can benefit you and others. As the field has begun to change, it is necessary that you change as well.

Adapt to the world of technology and use it to your advantage. Use the challenges that I have gone through as a way for you to advance. This new model of opportunity is suited directly to you. What you put in is what you will get out and through the Nurse Expert program, you are able to find a way to use the changes to the best of your ability. Make the possible negatives into positives and create the life for yourself that you desire.

By becoming a Nurse Expert, you are allowing yourself a number of opportunities at being your own boss, starting your own business and finding a career that suits you perfectly. It is a transition that is easy to make for any registered nurse, whether you have been working in the field for years, or just have graduated college, it is a step in the right direction. You have learned through this book the steps you need to take to find alternative careers in nursing.

Anyone Can Do it!

Imagine a mother of three who has been working as a registered bedside nurse day in and day out for 20 years. For her, the issue of supporting her family is what drove her to ignore the problems and negative aspects of her job. Her feelings were that she was overworked, underpaid and not nearly appreciated enough for all of the work that she put in. She would have told you that she would stay in those stressful and exhausting working conditions no matter what the circumstances, and that was what she did. That is until she found out about the opportunities that lay beyond the work of a bedside nurse.

As it became harder to leave the kids at home or at daycare in order to work, she searched for a way to continue to support her family and help others, while being there for her children more. The Nurse Expert was the perfect solution for her. She was able to learn about how to use her knowledge and experience in a way that allowed her to stay at home. She began writing articles and books about her work experience, and she learned how to become her own boss.

She was able to find ways to use her knowledge and a work schedule that allowed her the precious time with family that she so wanted while not incapacitating the need to support her family financially. At the age of forty and after twenty years in the nursing field, she was able to turn her life around and create the one that she had been dreaming of.

It is stories like these that inspire me and push me to continue to add to this program and find new ways to help registered nurses get out of their slump and into a career that means something more to them.

This is the beginning of a new life!

Take this information you have found in this book and apply it to your life. It is a transition that is easy for nurses to make and the benefits and opportunities are endless. You can gain control of your income, your work schedule and the love for your job. Take the chance to set yourself free from the chains of working for a corporation and learn the value of being able to work for yourself to be your own boss. The information within this book and the program information found on www.TheNurseExpert.com are all that you need to create a life and career that is meaningful and catered to you.

Enjoyed this book?

Visit us at www.TheNurseExpert.com

Because I want you to allow me to keep this conversation we've started going, I have a valuable gift there waiting for you!

About The Author

While Dwayne Adams has been an active and successful registered nurse for over a decade, working in critical care and other areas of the field, he is also an accomplished entrepreneur. Capitalizing on his nursing expertise, he combined it with his business skills to create a successful new enterprise.

Along with his nursing education, Adams earned a bachelor's degree in business administration in the area of marketing, as well as a master's degree in finance. This education outside of the nursing field has given him the added edge he needed in order to become a successful entrepreneur and lead his company from growth through expansion.

His first business-related endeavor was to bridge the gap between registered nurses and those who could benefit from working with a health and wellness coach. With this idea in mind, he created a whole new concept and coined the term "RN Health Coach." His business concept of registered nurses becoming health coaches has been well received, and many nurses around the country have followed his lead and benefited from his advice.

As a business-savvy registered nurse, Adams not only created a lucrative new career field for those in nursing, but has also used his skills, education and experience to help them to be successful entrepreneurs. He understands what it takes to build a business, market it, and sustain it long-term.

Given the state of health that people across the nation are currently in, Adams has shown his genius by creating the RN Heath Coach field. His passion for helping nurses to put their skills and education into use beyond the setting of a hospital bedside, combined with his entrepreneurial mindset, has created a lucrative field for registered nurses to enter.

He has developed a recipe for success that creates a win-win situation for all involved. Registered nurses get the pleasure of doing what they love – helping people – while those in the community who need health and wellness coaching get the most qualified coaches available.

Adams has a unique perspective on the business world, because of his nursing background. This allows him to actively pinpoint the most effective ways for RN Health Coaches to build, promote, and enjoy their new career field. He is an expert in the areas of nursing and health and wellness coaching, but also in marketing, finance, and business.

Resource Websites

www.RNHealthCoach.com

www.HealthCoachNursingJobs.com

www.PRHealthCareCommunications.com

www.MedicalMarketingSEO.com

www.TheNurseExpert.com

Other Titles

The Nurse Expert Vol. 1, Secrets to Being Your Own Publicist

ISBN: 978-0-9850033-1-9

The Nurse Expert vol. 2, How to use radio to position yourself as

the authority in your field.

ISBN: 978-0-9850033-0-2

The Nurse Expert vol. 3, Your 3 Step formula for success.

ISBN: 978-0-9850033-2-6

RN Health Coaching, Manual for Success

ISBN: 978-0-9850033-6-4

**30
DAYS**
of online RN Health Coach Training
ONLY $1 SPECIAL OFFER
www.HealthCoachNursingJobs.com
Use Special Code:BBBook

leverage your knowledge
THE NURSE
expert
a greater influence, impact & income

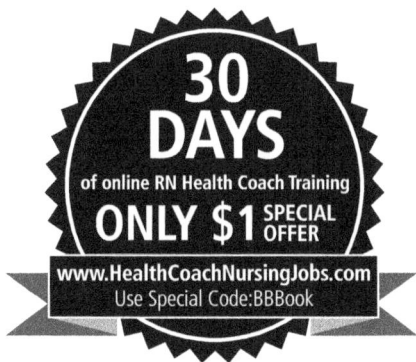

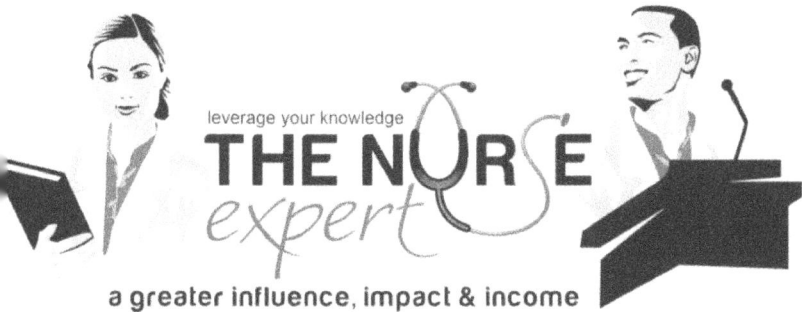

www.TheNurseExpert.com

www.ingramcontent.com/pod-product-compliance
Lightning Source LLC
Chambersburg PA
CBHW031957190326
41520CB00007B/281

* 9 7 8 0 9 8 5 0 0 3 3 3 3 *